The Ethics of Private Practice

The Ethics of Private Practice

*A Practical Guide for Mental
Health Clinicians*

BY JEFFREY E. BARNETT, PsyD, ABPP

JEFFREY ZIMMERMAN, PhD, ABPP

STEVEN WALFISH, PhD

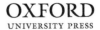

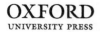

OXFORD
UNIVERSITY PRESS

Oxford University Press is a department of the University of
Oxford. It furthers the University's objective of excellence in research,
scholarship, and education by publishing worldwide.

Oxford   New York
Auckland   Cape Town   Dar es Salaam   Hong Kong   Karachi
Kuala Lumpur   Madrid   Melbourne   Mexico City   Nairobi
New Delhi   Shanghai   Taipei   Toronto

With offices in
Argentina   Austria   Brazil   Chile   Czech Republic   France   Greece
Guatemala   Hungary   Italy   Japan   Poland   Portugal   Singapore
South Korea   Switzerland   Thailand   Turkey   Ukraine   Vietnam

Oxford is a registered trademark of Oxford University Press
in the UK and certain other countries.

Published in the United States of America by
Oxford University Press
198 Madison Avenue, New York, NY 10016

Library of Congress Cataloging-in-Publication Data
Barnett, Jeffrey E., author.
The ethics of private practice : a practical guide for mental health clinicians / by Jeffrey E. Barnett,
Jeffrey Zimmerman, Steven Walfish.
   p. ; cm.
Includes bibliographical references and index.
ISBN 978-0-19-997662-1 (alk. paper)
I. Zimmerman, Jeffrey, author.   II. Walfish, Steven, author.   III. Title.
[DNLM: 1. Practice Management.   2. Psychology, Clinical.   3. Ethics, Clinical.
4. Mental Health Services—organization & administration.   5. Psychiatry. WM 21]
RC455.2.E8
174.2'9689—dc3
2014001804

To you the reader, to all recipients of mental health services, and to Stephanie, Lauren, and Mary, for their support of all we do.

CONTENTS

The world of private practice is full of risks and uncertainties for the mental health clinician. Due to the ever-changing nature of our field, it may seem almost impossible to keep up with ongoing developments and best practice standards clinically, ethically, and legally. Running a successful private practice brings with it the need for knowledge and skill in the business aspects of practice. Even the most clinically competent practitioner will find numerous business aspects of practice to be challenging. Further, many of the aspects of running a successful mental health practice carry a range of ethical and legal challenges and pitfalls. We have written this book as a practical guide to help you examine the way you practice and consider the many options for reducing the risk of ethical transgressions.

Throughout the book we speak to you as if you are sitting in front of us seeking a consultation. Rather than adopting a formal writing style, we have decided to be more user-friendly with the intent to make this book a practical guide that you can read from cover to cover and also come back to from time to time when you have a question related to a particular chapter or ethical dilemma. Each chapter can stand on its own. As such you will find certain concepts addressed in multiple chapters (e.g., confidentiality, collections activities, marketing). In some places the concept is touched on, and in others it is dealt with in far greater depth with recommendations being made pertinent to the particular chapter. We have also designed this book for people who are at all levels of practice, including those just starting out, those transitioning into solo practice (whether part time or full time), those who already have an established solo practice, and those who are looking to develop a group practice.

In looking at ethical transgressions, we believe that most violations occur as a function of a lack of situational awareness, rather than intentionally hurtful or deceitful behavior on the part of the clinician. That is, many factors conspire to increase the likelihood of the professional exercising poor judgment. Some of these factors are:

- The administrative structure of the office
- Suboptimal financial policies and procedures

- Failure to obtain truly informed consent from all those involved in treatment
- Documentation processes that are lacking
- The need for protocols for sharing information with third parties and dealing with high-pressure requests for information
- How one supervises professional and administrative staff
- Marketing and advertising activities
- The need for a commitment to ongoing professional development and self-care
- Pressure that we feel to respond quickly in a situation

Certainly, although any one of these areas and others can lead to an ethical breach, the more risks that are present at one time the greater the likelihood that such a problem will occur.

Throughout this book we will address some issues that you may think relate more to the law than to ethics. There is a strong interaction between the two, such that behaviors that are illegal (e.g., fraudulent) are also unethical. Additionally, some of the requirements of the law (e.g., requests for documents) can put the clinician in an ethical conundrum, where in certain situations complying or not complying with a request can lead to charges of unethical conduct. In the following pages we address many places where the law and ethics converge.

Each chapter has a discussion of the common issues at hand with recommendations included in the text. We identify key risks and then practical options to address these risks with the goal of helping you decrease your vulnerability to inadvertent ethical pitfalls. Each chapter also includes specific lists of ethical challenges, key points to keep in mind, practical recommendations, and pitfalls to avoid, followed by a sampling of some pertinent ethical requirements (from multiple professional ethics codes) and references. The chapters also relate to one another, and you will see certain concepts introduced in one chapter and expanded in another.

We begin in Chapter 1 by addressing the issues you will likely confront when starting out in practice. Chapter 2 then focuses on the broader issues of clinical practice at any stage of one's career. Chapters 3 and 4 address the ethical issues related to documentation, record keeping, dealing with third party requests for information, and protecting confidentiality.

Chapters 5, 6, and 7 focus on the ethics issues relevant to the business of practice as we address ethics challenges and practices in areas such as the financial elements of practice, dealing with administrative and clinical staff, and advertising and marketing. Chapters 8 and 9 then get more focused on you, your professional development, self-care, and eventually leaving active practice. Thus, we take you through the lifespan of your practice, in different environments and from clinical, business, and personal perspectives.

One fundamental concept emphasized throughout the book is our belief that excellence in care comes from a convergence of factors that many people think are in conflict. We believe that the healthiest and most helpful practices provide the best clinical care that mental health clinicians can provide (something that changes over the course of one's career as skills develop and fade), in an environment that operates based on sound business and ethical practice principles. These are not in conflict. We believe they actually support each other and are required to reliably reach the highest level of service delivery, while appropriately protecting both you and your clients (please note that the terms *client* and *patient* are used interchangeably throughout this book).

We hope this book will serve as a valuable resource that you will come back to time and time again as you work to develop the most effective, ethical, and legal private practice possible, and as you integrate the suggestions and recommendations provided in these chapters into your day-to-day business of practice activities. We hope you find this book to be thought provoking and that it will help you confirm that you are on the right track in many areas, giving you pause to consider options in others. If at some point in your reading you stop and say, "Gee, I didn't think of that," then we've done our job.

Jeffrey E. Barnett, PsyD, ABPP
Jeffrey Zimmerman, PhD, ABPP
Steven Walfish, PhD

ACKNOWLEDGMENTS

We are deeply grateful to Sarah Harrington and Andrea Zekus of Oxford University Press for their active encouragement and ongoing support throughout each phase of the process, from helping us to develop our ideas into a detailed book proposal, to taking our initial drafts and assisting us in developing them into this book that we are so proud of. Further, we express our thanks to the production team at Oxford University Press, Emily Perry and James Fraleigh, as well as Andrea Guinn for the excellent cover design. Finally, we thank all our colleagues who have helped to shape our ideas and whose generous consultations have added to our expertise.

The Ethics of Private Practice

Starting Out

Ethics Issues in Beginning a Practice

Starting a private practice can be overwhelming for the new mental health professional. There are both clinical and business skills to learn in order to be successful in private practice. Additionally, ethics and legal considerations must be addressed if you are to develop an effective and sustained private practice. In this chapter we address the ethics and legal issues related to becoming licensed as a professional, supervision prior to licensure, choosing a practice, and practicing in integrated healthcare settings.

BECOMING LICENSED TO PRACTICE

Much to the chagrin of many a graduate student and early career professional, it takes a long time to become licensed to practice independently as a mental health professional. In medicine a physician may become licensed quickly upon graduation from medical school. By contrast, before you can become licensed in psychology there are many rungs to climb while going up the career ladder. First, you have to obtain a doctorate. On average this takes 5 to 6 years, including internship. Then, in most jurisdictions, you have to complete a postdoctoral year of training. This is typically 1,500 to 2,000 hours in length. It may be completed in formal settings such as a university medical school, college counseling center, or a paid position in an agency or organization in which a licensed psychologist will provide the necessary supervision. This requirement may also be satisfied in an informal setting, such as a group private practice. Read the regulations in your jurisdiction carefully, as some jurisdictions have specific requirements about how many hours of supervision are required, in what venues (individual vs. group), and by whom (i.e., whether or not you can purchase supervision and whether the supervisor has to be a full-time employee of the facility). Other factors are the length of time the supervisor has been licensed and type of license.

To become licensed as a psychologist, you also have to earn a passing score on the Examination for Professional Practice in Psychology. Jurisdictions vary in when they will allow the prospective licensee to take this exam. Some allow this prior to completing all doctoral requirements, and others prior to completing all postdoctoral requirements. This exam focuses on knowledge of eight content areas in psychology in general, not specifically on clinical or counseling psychology (see http://www.asppb.net and click on EPPP Applicants/Students and then on Info for Candidates). Once a passing score is achieved based on the cutoff score for the jurisdiction in which you are seeking licensure, there are additional exams that must be passed. Their number and type vary by jurisdiction. Most jurisdictions have an exam that focuses on laws and regulations that govern the practice of psychology in that jurisdiction. This may include questions regarding required record keeping, involuntary hospitalization (the procedure to hospitalize clients who are a danger to themselves or others varies by jurisdiction), whether there is a "duty to warn" or "duty to protect" law in that jurisdiction (Werth, Welfel, & Benjamin, 2008; see also Chapter 2, "Dangerousness and Exceptions to Confidentiality"), and ethics, among a variety of other questions regarding practice in the particular jurisdiction. In addition, some jurisdictions then require an oral examination in which an applicant for licensure may present a case to a group of psychologists who will evaluate his or her competence to practice. Some jurisdictions (e.g., New York) also require the applicant to take an online course in child protection issues and procedures. See http://www.asppb.org/HandbookPublic/before.aspx for a list of examination requirements for psychology licensure in each jurisdiction.

As can be seen from the preceding, although it may take a psychology graduate student 5 to 6 years to obtain a doctorate, it may take another 1 to 2 years until you can become licensed to practice independently (i.e., without supervision) and call yourself a "psychologist." The education required for licensure in social work, professional counseling, and marriage and family therapy is typically less time intensive, because the entry-level degree is a master's degree. This varies, however, as many jurisdictions require 60 graduate credits to be eligible for licensure as a professional counselor rather then the typical 48-credit master's degree. Additionally, the supervised work experience for these professions is typically longer than for psychology, because psychology graduate students may accrue many more supervised clinical hours during their externships during the 4 or more years in their doctoral program and the yearlong internship they must complete.

From an ethical and legal standpoint, it is essential that those desiring to become licensed know and understand the statutory requirements. Each jurisdiction's licensing board posts this information on its website; it may also be obtained directly from the government department that oversees the practice of the profession within the jurisdiction (e.g., Board of Social Work). It is crucial to know whether licensure requires graduation from a program that meets specific accreditation requirements. For example, in psychology a few jurisdictions require graduation from an American Psychological Association (APA)–approved training program. Other jurisdictions may allow for graduation from a program deemed

"APA-approved equivalent." However, the burden is placed on the licensure applicant to document this equivalency. It is up to the applicant in all of the mental health fields to provide the necessary documentation that all requirements have been satisfied. As such, we suggest becoming an expert in the statutes governing practice in the jurisdiction in which you plan to become licensed, so that you can prepare properly during training. The importance of this suggestion should not be overlooked when planning your graduate education. For instance, some licensure boards may require you to complete specific courses. Thus, knowing the specific licensure requirements in your jurisdiction from the outset can influence the education and training experiences you select.

It also is wise to become familiar with the relevant statutes in any jurisdiction in which you think you might want to reside at a later date. For example, if you did your training in Wyoming and your family lives in Florida, and one day you want to live close to your family, then you should review the statute for practice in your discipline in Florida as well. This will help reduce the likelihood that you will have difficulties with licensure mobility. Knowing what is required in the jurisdictions where you may want to practice also can affect your selection of degree options, the courses you choose to take during training, and the amount of supervised clinical experience you complete.

ACCURACY AND INTEGRITY IN COMPLETING LICENSURE APPLICATIONS

This may sound like a no-brainer, but from an ethical and legal perspective it is important when you fill out applications for licensure that you "tell the truth, the whole truth, and nothing but the truth." Licensure applications are not a place to embellish or exaggerate your qualifications. Indeed, most applications include a statement at the end indicating that providing false information on a licensure application constitutes a felony.

In addition to basic information such as demographic data, places of education, and degrees obtained, most licensure applications will also ask personal information, such as: Have you ever been arrested? Have you ever been treated for alcohol or drug abuse? Have you ever been treated for a mental disorder? Such questions may seem highly personal and, in your belief system, to be "nobody's business" but your own. However, you are ethically and legally responsible to answer these questions truthfully. The purpose of licensure is to protect the public. Whether it is good, bad, or indifferent that you have previously been treated for an alcohol problem, the licensing board has decided that it has a right to know this in making the decision to grant you the privilege to practice in their jurisdiction.

In our opinion, these questions are not asked to prevent you from practicing. Rather, they are used to inform the jurisdiction that this has previously been an issue and to allow you to provide documentation to demonstrate that it is no longer a problem area. It is especially important to be truthful just in case at a later date there is a relapse, such as drinking again. The licensure board may then prefer that you participate in a treatment and monitoring program for impaired professionals as a way to protect the public and allow you to continue practicing once this is no longer an active problem. On the other hand, if they later discover that you had committed a felony by lying or omitting essential information on your initial application, this is typically considered grounds for the board to revoke your license to practice.

It is imperative that in the process of applying for licensure, you are explicitly clear that you have answered questions about the type and amount of postgraduate clinical hours, number of supervisors, and amount of supervision, as well as the relationship of your supervisor(s) to you and the postdoctoral facility, with the utmost care toward accurate reporting. This is as important as the representations about your training we mentioned previously. Mental health professionals have to engage in postgraduate training, have this work supervised, and then provide documentation of this training before they can even make an application for licensure in their jurisdiction. This points to the importance of recording and maintaining accurate records of all supervised clinical experience throughout your training.

SUPERVISION PRIOR TO LICENSURE

Supervised experience may be obtained in a work setting or through a formal internship or fellowship program. The number of hours of supervised work experience required for licensure is determined by each individual jurisdiction, and these requirements are delineated in the jurisdiction's statutes or regulations. A few jurisdictions have eliminated the postdoctoral requirements of an additional year of supervised clinical experience for licensure for psychologists. However, because not all jurisdictions have done so, it may become problematic if the psychologist practicing in one jurisdiction wants to move to another jurisdiction that does have the postdoctoral training/supervision requirement. For example, Washington State does not have this postdoctoral requirement, but California does. If at a later date a psychologist licensed in Washington wants to move to California to practice, the California Board of Psychology may not recognize their Washington license. They would then have to complete the required supervised postdoctoral work experience before being allowed to be licensed in California, regardless of how long the person had practiced in Washington—whether it be 5, 10, or 20 years or longer. The safest way to assure this will not be an issue is to have a year of supervised work experience postlicensure even if it is not required in the jurisdiction granting the original license.

What is supervision? Bernard and Goodyear (2014) indicate that a significant amount of variability exists in the literature in defining this activity and responsibility. However, they describe that supervision focuses on legal, ethical, and professional issues, citing literature in which the supervisor takes legal and professional responsibility for the work of the supervisee. Thus the clinical activities of the supervisee become the legal responsibility of the supervisor. In our view of supervision, a more senior, experienced, and expert professional accepts responsibility for the clinical services the subordinate provides, and also offers clinical oversight and training, to promote the supervisee's professional growth and development.

Thomas (2010) points out that informed consent is an important issue in the psychotherapist–client relationship. Ethically, providing adequate informed consent recognizes the autonomy of the client in respecting his or her right to decide whether or not to enter into a psychotherapy relationship. Clients should know the nature of the relationship, what is likely to take place in treatment, what fees are involved, and what happens if the treatment does not go well. In this vein, Thomas argues that informed consent for entering into a supervisory relationship is equally as important as when entering a psychotherapy relationship. She presents a table of informed consent supervision issues between supervisor and supervisee that are addressed in each of the mental health professions' ethics codes. These include: (a) supervisor privacy; (b) job duties and required experiences; (c) supervisor's credentials or orientation; (d) due process for supervisees; (e) supervision boundaries, multiple relationships, exploitation, and power; (f) documentation of consent; (g) evaluation; (h) required self-disclosure and personal growth activities; (i) fees; (j) conditions of supervision; (k) client privacy in supervision; and (l) disclosure of trainee status. Not all of the mental health professions emphasize each of these, but it is noteworthy that supervision has a prominent place in ethics codes.

For example, many years ago, one of us in our private practice was co-supervising a postdoctoral resident. The other supervisor was another partner in the practice. One day the supervisee was told that the co-supervisors were discussing a particular issue from a recent supervision session. The supervisee became upset, asking, "Whatever happened to confidentiality in supervision?" The immediate response was, "There is no inherent confidentiality in supervision. If you would like for there to be, then we can discuss putting that into place, but until we agree on it there is no confidentiality." A mutual understanding regarding confidentiality was then reached. The important thing to understand is that there had been a misunderstanding regarding this issue that was quite important to the supervisee and potentially damaging to the supervisory alliance and the level of trust in this relationship. If the nature of confidentiality of the supervisory relationship had been discussed and agreed upon from the beginning, this could have been avoided and there would have been no surprise.

It is important that the supervisor and supervisee develop a supervision contract at the outset of the professional relationship. Such a document provides a framework for the expectations and responsibilities of each party and outlines the nature of what is to take place during supervision. Thomas (2010) provides guidance for what information might be included in a supervision contract.

Barnett (2000) presents a checklist for ethical and legal considerations in the supervision process. An adaptation of this checklist for supervisees is presented in Table 1.1. These issues focus on assessment of competence, informed consent, confidentiality, the nature of the relationship between supervisor and supervisee

Table 1.1 THE SUPERVISEE'S CHECKLIST

1. Supervisee Competence: Supervisors should assess supervisee training needs and competence to determine the nature and extent of additional training and supervision needed.
2. Supervisor Competence: Supervisors should only supervise in those areas of practice where they are competent.
3. Informed Consent: Supervisors should utilize a comprehensive informed consent process at the beginning of the supervisory relationship.
4. Supervision as a Safety Zone: The supervisory process should feel safe, not threatening or punitive.
5. Paranoia vs. Trust: Ensure that both the level and intensity of supervision are adequate for your training needs.
6. Accurate Representation: Be sure you represent and advertise yourself in a manner that does not imply competence or licensure that you do not have.
7. Limits to Confidentiality: Ensure that informed consent agreements with patients address the limits to confidentiality to include your supervisor's involvement in the treatment process.
8. Documentation: In addition to thorough documentation of clinical services provided, be sure both you and your supervisor document the supervisory sessions to include any recommendations made or issues for you to follow up on with patients.
9. Legal and Ethics Issues: Be sure that thorough attention is paid to legal and ethics issues in supervision in addition to patient treatment issues.
10. Diversity Issues: Supervisors should be sensitive to diversity issues between themselves and you as well as with regard to each patient's treatment.
11. Boundary Issues and Multiple Relationships: In addition to all issues typically considered in relationships with patients, supervisors and supervisees must be sensitive to the fine line that at times exists between supervision and psychotherapy.
12. Consultation: When unsure about any of these or related issues, consult with an experienced colleague.
13. The Supervisee as Professional: Remember the serious professional obligation you have to your patients, to your supervisor, and to the profession. Take your training seriously and keep in mind the great impact you have on your patients' lives.

Adapted from "The Supervisee's Checklist: Ethical, Legal, and Clinical Issues," by J. E. Barnett, 2000, *The Maryland Psychologist, 4,* 18–20. Used with permission of the author.

and the need to develop trust, the importance of documentation, legal and ethics issues, and diversity issues.

It is important to be cognizant of individual jurisdictions' licensing boards' laws and regulations regarding supervision. For example, in some jurisdictions supervisors within a private practice setting are precluded from charging the supervisee fees for the supervision, whereas in other jurisdictions supervisors may charge fees. Ethically, it may be viewed as a conflict of interest to have a situation in which the supervisee pays for supervision and the supervisor in turn has to evaluate and vouch for their ability to practice independently. In some ways this is like an employer (the supervisee) paying an employee or consultant (the supervisor) who is in a position to evaluate the person paying them for the service. Thomas (2010) states, "Supervisors and psychotherapists alike must be vigilant to ensure that their need for business does not lead to their becoming inappropriately accommodating or to avoid confronting problematic behavior so as to dodge conflict" (p. 112).

Where the supervisor and supervisee are required to be located may vary from jurisdiction to jurisdiction. For example, in some jurisdictions it is required that the supervisor always be colocated in the same practice or facility as the supervisee, being physically present whenever the supervisee is providing clinical services in case an emergency or crisis with a client occurs. In other jurisdictions this may not be a requirement. The amount of supervision required per week or month may also vary by jurisdiction, as may the number of clients seen per week. Someone seeing 10 clients per week may not require as much supervision as someone seeing 30 clients per week. All such expectations must be made clear from the outset and should be agreed to in the supervision contract. It is each supervisee's responsibility to ensure that these requirements are met. It would be most unfortunate to be informed by the licensure board reviewing your licensure application that you did not receive enough hours of supervision (or clinical experience) to qualify for licensure. Thus, precise monitoring to actively ensure that all licensure requirements are met is an important responsibility for each supervisee to attend to throughout each aspect of training.

It is also important to periodically review the adequacy of the contract to ensure that supervision is adequate in terms of content and time to meet the training needs of the supervisee and the clinical needs of the clients. For example, there may be a statute that indicates that 1 hour of supervision must take place for every 10 clinical hours provided. However, a supervisee (or supervisor) may not find this frequency of supervision adequate to ensure that competent clinical work is taking place with clients being treated, especially if they are working with a complicated treatment population. In such cases there is an ethical obligation for both supervisee and supervisor to revisit this part of the contract. It is important to understand that supervision requirements in statutes are only minimal expectations that must be met to be in compliance with the law. Good clinical judgment dictates, however, that we each receive the needed supervision to ensure that our clients' clinical needs are met.

From an ethical and legal perspective, it is important that the supervisee does not misrepresent their status as a professional. For example, in Georgia, prior to licensure counselors may only refer to themselves as Associate Licensed Professional Counselors. Similarly, there is a designation as an Associate Marriage and Family Therapist for those in that field. Those with doctorates in psychology pursuing licensure must refer to themselves as "psychology residents" in some jurisdictions and as "psychology associates" in others. As part of the informed consent process in client disclosure forms, those not licensed to practice independently must ethically and legally inform their clients of their training status and also provide the name of the licensed professional who is providing clinical supervision and taking responsibility for their work. There are prospective applicants who have pended applications for licensure (not a good thing) because they are being investigated for practicing without a license when, as an unlicensed professional, they or their employer used terms and descriptions on websites that are only appropriate for licensed professionals. Thus, care should be taken in how you represent yourself to the public, only using professional titles allowed by law based on your level of training and your licensure status. Do not just presume that your supervisor knows the correct description to use. One of the authors was misinformed during his postdoctoral year by his supervisor and received a call from the chair of the licensing board notifying him that he was misrepresenting himself. Calls like that can be quite upsetting and problematic.

Supervisees must also ensure that their supervisor is skilled in the relevant area of practice to provide supervision of their work. This is because the licensed professional is taking responsibility for their clinical work (Bernard & Goodyear, 2014). Supervisors who are not clinically competent in particular areas of practice cannot ethically and legally provide supervision of others practicing in these clinical areas. Supervisees, as part of the informed consent process, should learn the areas of expertise of their supervisor. Barnett (2007) states, "Modeling ethical and professional behavior along with emphasizing a focus on ethical practice throughout the supervisory process are additional and essential qualities of effective supervisors" (p. 270). Licensed mental health professionals have an ethical responsibility not to practice outside of the scope of their expertise and clinical competence.

In the co-supervising example cited earlier, the postdoctoral resident had two supervisors because he provided clinical services to different client populations. He saw children and adolescents as well as adults. One of the supervisors did not have expertise in child and adolescent psychology. Had that person supervised the trainee's work in this area, the supervisor would have been practicing outside of his or her areas of expertise, and the supervisee would have been (a) practicing outside of his area of expertise and (b) provided with inadequate supervision. So, one of the psychologists supervised the psychology resident's child and adolescent work of and the other the adult work. This further reinforces the importance of every supervisee's training needs being assessed at the beginning of the supervisory relationship so that appropriate supervision can be provided and appropriate training experiences designed.

Supervisees must also understand that not all of their training and professional development needs may be met within one setting or with one supervisor. Some jurisdictions may actually require that there be more than one supervisor. Although not specifically applicable for licensure purposes, we think it is beneficial that those beginning their careers adopt a mindset of seeking out further consultation and training from competent professionals, even if they have to pay for these services. This mindset is part of the lifelong learning that will serve all professionals well throughout their careers.

For those of us who are supervisors, occasionally we may supervise someone who asks us to "fudge" hours or who is functioning in an ethically questionably manner. Each supervisor has a responsibility to confront the supervisee and make sure that he or she is not functioning in a way that will put patients (or the supervisor's license to practice) at risk. This can be especially difficult as none of us want to be the individual that impedes someone's ability to become licensed after a long course of study. Yet our responsibility to the community and our profession, as well as to the supervisee, comes before doing what the supervisee wants or will be easier in the short run. It is important to keep careful records of the dates and amount of supervision provided as well as the key issues discussed during the supervision session (as you would if you were providing direct clinical care).

There also may be times when a licensed professional is learning new skills and asks that you "supervise" their work if you are an expert in that particular area. There is a major distinction between "supervision" and "consultation." When you agree to be a supervisor, you are in essence accepting responsibility for the clinical work of the supervisee. This should not be done unless this is your specific intention. Often, when another licensed professional requests "supervision," they are really asking for peer consultation. Consultation is a service provided by one licensed professional to another. It is up to the individual seeking the consultation to make his or her own decisions about what to do with the consultation provided, and the consultant takes no responsibility for the professional services provided (Barnett, 2013). This distinction should be made clear and agreed upon by both parties from the start.

CHOOSING A PRACTICE

Once licensed and entering private practice, most individuals choose to practice either on their own as a solo practitioner or as part of a group practice. With a group of mental health practitioners this may take the form of an actual corporate structure. However, many mental health professionals decide to practice together in the same setting, but do not develop a formal group or legal structure. They are just clinicians practicing in the same space and sharing professional expenses. In some instances there will be practice owners who invite clinicians to join the practice, and this relationship may be as a salaried employee, associate, partner, or as an independent contractor.

In terms of ethical considerations, there are pros and cons of practicing on one's own as well as practicing in a group setting. Whether formally or informally structured, the strength of a group practice is that you are practicing in the same setting as other mental health professionals. This allows for ready access to these professionals to discuss cases or issues formally or informally when an ethical dilemma arises. In addition, it is difficult to remain current on changes in laws and the thinking on ethics issues. Being around other professionals may increase the likelihood that discussion about these issues will take place as just a normal part of working in the same setting (e.g., "Did you see that article in the last issue of *Professional Psychology* on storing your records in the cloud?"). Being in a group practice setting also helps to combat the effects of professional isolation that may occur when one is a solo practitioner. Interacting with colleagues informally can help reduce the risk of burnout developing, a condition that can easily have an adverse impact on one's clinical competence.

If you decide to be a solo practitioner, it is important that you arrange your professional life so that although you may be practicing alone, you do not practice in isolation. Handelsman (2001) suggests that without input from other mental health professionals, a clinician is at risk of becoming too insulated, too narrow in their thinking, and hence at increased risk for unethical conduct. So, if you do practice alone, we think it important to ensure that you will have input from other clinicians. Ways to obtain this input may include but not be limited to such activities as (a) joining a consultation group with a senior clinician leading the group, (b) participating in a peer consultation group that meets one or two times per month and where cases (without identifying information) are discussed, (c) meeting with a senior clinician individually one or two times per month for case consultation (as opposed to supervision, as the senior clinician will not be taking responsibility for the case), and (d) participating on the ethics committee of your jurisdiction's professional organization. In addition, the major malpractice carriers have risk management consultants available by appointment to consult about cases in which an ethical or legal question may arise. The carriers make this service available as a way to help guide clinicians who may want input or confirmation about how to respond to an issue. Questions such as, "How do I respond to this subpoena that I just received?" and "The noncustodial parent of the child I am seeing wants to see my treatment notes, so do I provide them?" are common occurrences that arise in practice. It is important to have risk managers available for consultation to help ensure that you are following proper legal and ethical procedures. It is a service that you pay for with your insurance premium, so make use of it whenever you feel the need. The carrier is happy to provide this service as it also reduces the risk of a malpractice claim being filed against you. It is also very important to document in the patient record these discussions and all other consultations that occur on a case.

If you decide to practice in a group setting, it is important to choose your new colleagues wisely, from a business, clinical, and ethics perspective. Woody (2013) points out that a clinician may be held liable for the misdeeds of others working in the office, both professionals and support staff. According to Woody, "A mental health professional is known by the company that he or she keeps. If there is a shared enterprise the 'innocent' practitioner may have legal (vicarious or imputed) liability" (p. 90). Walfish and Barnett (2009) present a long series of questions a clinician could consider asking when evaluating a group practice to join. Several of these questions relate to ethics issues. Most early-career professionals, when interviewing with a practice, usually conceptualize this as a one-way interview (i.e., "Can I impress them enough to get them to ask me to join the practice?"). We think it important to conceptualize this as a two-way interview, including having a mindset question, such as, "Is this a practice that I would want to join?"

In addition to evaluating clinical and business aspects of the practice, ethics issues should be in the forefront of your mind as well. Ask if any members of the practice have ever had complaints filed against them with the jurisdiction's licensing board, and if so, what the charges and outcomes were. Ask if any have had malpractice suits filed against them and the outcome of each case. When interviewing, clinicians are often asked a simple question: "Describe to me an ethical dilemma that you encountered and how you resolved it." The purpose of the question is to see how the clinician thinks about difficult ethical situations. However, we think it would be equally reasonable to ask the person (or persons) doing the interview the same question. In this way you may get a sense of the ethical decision making of those working in the practice. As Woody (2013) noted, you may be held vicariously liable for the behavior of those in your practice. In short, one question to ask yourself is, "Is this group composed of individuals who have established a culture that I would like to be part of?" When one of the authors was being recruited to join a practice, he asked the practice owner whether there was any peer consultation on cases and was told, "That's not needed in my practice. I just hire good people." This led to the applicant pulling out of the process, as he did not want to affiliate with a practice that did not invest in professional development and ethical risk-management activities for its professional employees.

If you practice in a group setting, assurances must be made regarding confidentiality of your clients' records. Policies and procedures must be put in place and reviewed prior to joining the practice, and these should be stated in a written agreement. Who will have access to your files? This should be you and support staff as needed to carry out administrative tasks (e.g., billing and collecting, sending records after a properly obtained authorization has been received and reviewed by the practitioner). Are your files commingled with the files of clients of the other practitioners in the office, or are they kept in a separate locked cabinet that only you and your support staff can access? We recommend the latter. Who has access to your voice mail and e-mails? We suggest following the advice of Fisher (2009), who recommends finding out whether the office staff has been adequately trained in issues related to ethics and protection of clients. (See Chapters 3 and 6 for further discussion of these issues). We suggest inquiring about what the training has been and if the standards taught to the administrative staff are at a level that meets your own standards. Administrative staff members are your representatives and thus you are accountable for their actions, even if you are in a group practice and do not have administrative authority over other staff members.

In a similar vein, it is important to review the practice's billing and collection procedures during the interview process. Although these tasks may be delegated to an administrative employee or an outside billing agency, the mental health practitioner is still responsible for the actions of these individuals. If a client does not pay the fees that are due, does the practice have a policy of turning the account over to a collection agency? We suggest not, but if such a policy is set in place by the practice, can you opt out of this policy? What occurs if an insurance carrier denies a claim due to a diagnosis that they deem not reimbursable? Does the office staff simply (and inappropriately) change the diagnosis to fit one that will be reimbursed, or is this brought to the attention of the clinician to decide how to proceed? These are examples of questions related to ethical responsibilities that mental health professionals should ask about the billing and collection procedures of the practice they may be joining. These important points and related administrative practices will be discussed in far more detail in other chapters.

PRACTICING IN HEALTH CARE SETTINGS

There is a significant movement toward integrating mental health care into medical health care settings. Nordal (2012) sees a role for mental health professionals who can successfully adapt their style of practice to fit what is needed in a health care setting. Runyan (2011) provides a rationale for mental health professionals to be involved in patient-centered medical homes. Given the mind–body connection in the development and maintenance of medical problems, there is a natural role for clinicians to practice alongside medical professionals. Indeed, it makes sense that if you want to work with children, you should rent space in a busy pediatrician's office, rather than join a mental health practice. If you have a specialty in working with women's issues, then rent space in an OB-GYN practice. If you treat chronic pain, consider renting space in an orthopedic surgery or rehabilitation medicine practice. Kelly and Coons (2012) present a list of books helpful for mental health professionals interested in learning more about working in primary care.

Reiter and Runyan (2013) suggest that those whose only professional experience has been in the traditional mental health care system will be surprised about the frequent occurrence of ethical issues that arise in a primary care setting. This is due to the complexity of relationships in health care settings compared to the solo practice setting for the mental health professional. A number of legal and ethics issues should be considered when a mental health professional works as an independent tenant (as opposed to being an employee) in such a setting. Coons and Gablis (2010) discuss such issues in cases when a private practitioner colocates his or her practice in a medical setting. Regarding the contractual agreement, they state:

> While the final content of agreements will likely vary, most should address the following issues: 1) the term of the agreement and grounds for termination; 2) the cost and schedule for use of the space; 3) patient referrals; 4) insurance coverage(s) and documentation; 5) confidentiality of patient records and propriety matters; 6) storage and ownership of patient records; 7) use of office resources; and 8) marketing concerns. (p. 181)

It is important to be sensitive to the process around receiving referrals. The mental health professional may colocate a practice with the hope of receiving referrals from the health care providers to whom they are paying rent. However, it would be unethical for the person or organization renting the space to guarantee a certain number of referrals to the mental health clinician. They need to be free to refer to any provider who will best meet their patients' needs, and at times this may not be the mental health professional in their office. Similarly, the clinician cannot base the amount of rent they pay to the practice on the number of referrals received, or this may be considered paying for referrals. Rent should be based on the space, time utilized, and administrative services the landlord provides, not on the number of referrals.

When separate practices are colocated in a setting, it is essential that, prior to communicating with another health care provider about a client, you must almost always first receive written permission to do so, even though the physician referred the client in the first place. This is easily done at the outset of treatment. Even if you are employed by the medical practice, the consent to treatment can specify that the referring physician and treating mental health professional may exchange information (this can help avoid a sense of betrayal and inappropriate expectations on the part of the client). If you are a separate legal entity you can have the client specifically sign a release allowing the exchange of information. In either case, this should be explicitly discussed with, and agreed upon by, the client in advance of the communication.

Hudgins, Rose, Fifield, and Arnault (2013) discuss the issues of both confidentiality and informed consent when mental health professionals are practicing in a medical setting. They review legal influences on confidentiality and informed consent including the Health Insurance Portability and Accountability Act of 1996 (HIPAA), federal rules, state law, and case law. They note that "consent to exchange or release information between primary care providers and behavioral health professionals has proven to be cumbersome, requiring cross-training, and a great deal of compromise" (p. 10). For example, they point out that in traditional mental health practices it is not difficult for the clinician to provide full informed consent prior to initiating assessment or treatment services. In their review they found that this may not be as easy to achieve in an integrated care setting. We recommend that prior to practicing in a medical setting, mental health clinicians review the complex issues put forth by Hudgins et al. (2013). Physicians and mental health professionals do not share the same ethics codes or practice patterns, and it is essential that the potential differences be discussed proactively, rather than reactively.

Coons and Gablis (2010) note that when colocated in a medical practice, the mental health professional needs to maintain treatment records separately from the regular medical record. This is because the mental health professional is an independent practitioner and not an employee of the practice. Even if the mental health professional is employed by the practice, it still might make sense to keep separate records, given the potential for there to be highly confidential information in the file to which other staff should not have easy access. As there is greater movement toward use of electronic health records, this may change, but confidentiality is an issue to attend to closely in integrated settings, as changes take place in record-keeping requirements for mental health records. Along the same lines, Coons and Gablis (2010) indicate that storage and retention of the client's mental health record is the obligation of the mental health professional, and not the medical practice.

As part of the complexity of colocating in a medical practice, if you are an effective clinician, staff working in the practice may want to seek out your services. Kanzler, Goodie, Hunter, Glotfelter, and Bodart (2013) present a scenario in which a physician in the practice wants the clinician to be their own personal psychotherapist. These authors discuss issues related to multiple relationships, informed consent, and confidentiality in such an instance. Can you maintain objectivity with someone who is a referral source for you? How might it impact relationships with other practitioners in the clinic? As part of the health care team, might you serve on committees or work on projects together? How these possible scenarios may impact both direct clinical practice and ethical behavior should be considered prior to deciding if you will be seeing this colleague for psychotherapy. Kanzler et al. (2013) point to the importance of treating the colleague just like any other client in terms of providing them with the same informed consent procedures and paperwork, and maintenance of clinical records. They emphasize the importance of clarifying your role at the beginning of treatment, determining the risks and benefits of being the behavioral health provider for this physician, and discussing concerns about being able to maintain confidentiality in the setting.

Along these same lines, you may be asked to provide guidance for family members of those working in the clinic or to provide mental health information: "My son is being bullied in school, what do you recommend?" "My dad is starting to have problems with his memory, what should I do?" Providing general mental health information, referrals to practitioners who specialize in the problem area, or directing them to books on the topic all fall in the purview of being a "good citizen" in the office. However, care must be taken regarding becoming overinvolved and taking on a professional role in helping them resolve the problem. First, the issues of boundaries and multiple relationships previously mentioned are relevant to these situations. Second, although it may be tempting to give clinical advice in an effort to be helpful, without having evaluated the individual in question, you cannot competently provide clinical advice or recommendations.

YOUR ETHICS AND LEGAL TEAM

Due to convenience, and due to there being no cost, many mental health professionals will post questions related to mental health law, ethics, business of practice, and accounting on electronic mailing lists or listservs. Although these resources can provide useful information, they are not the same as seeking out professional advice and direction. One of the "Principles of Private Practice Success" presented by Walfish and Barnett (2009) states, "It is essential for mental health professionals to have ready access to competent professionals to answer questions outside of their area of expertise. Ignoring this principle places the clinician at ethical, legal, and financial risk" (p. 82). It does not make sense to obtain legal advice from a clinical social worker when it can be obtained from an attorney. Similarly, it does not make sense to obtain tax advice from a psychologist when a CPA is readily available for consultation. It also doesn't make sense to have a like professional give you well-meaning advice based on their experience and knowledge, which may not be applicable in the jurisdiction in which you practice. You may be provided with misinformation about an important issue.

As business-of-practice experts, we have often scratched our heads when reading advice offered on electronic mailing lists (e.g., "If you need to look professional when seeing clients you can write off the money that you spend on clothing on your taxes"). It is also important to have a professional take some accountability or responsibility for the advice or consultation provided to you. You cannot call in the person who offered tax advice on a listserv to advocate for you in an IRS audit. However, you can call in your CPA. You cannot bring in a colleague to argue with a licensing board about why you decided to warn or not warn a potential victim of violence. However, you can bring your attorney who specializes in mental health law to such a hearing to advocate on your behalf.

Although this principle is important if you are in a group practice, it is even more important if you are working in a solo practice. For this reason we think it essential that clinicians in independent practice invest in consultation time with: (a) an attorney familiar with mental health law and private practice issues, (b) a CPA, (c) a billing expert if you are doing third-party (e.g., insurance) billing, and (d) a senior mental health clinician or mentor who is willing to provide advice and guidance on clinical and practice issues. These individuals will increase the likelihood that you do not make ethical transgressions or break the law and can help you plan and problem-solve around important and difficult practice issues.

You do not need to have an attorney on retainer, but prior to opening your practice it is important to develop a relationship with an attorney. Do so ahead of time, because it is not a matter of if you will ever need to consult with a mental health attorney, but rather when and how often. Do not wait until you are faced with a legal question in your practice before searching for an attorney to know how to properly respond as a professional. Take these two examples:

1. You have received a valid request for treatment records from the executor of the estate for a client who recently died. Can you release this record?
2. The parent of a 15-year old client wants you to tell the secrets you have been told in psychotherapy sessions. Do you legally have to honor this request?

The answer to these questions may depend on the jurisdiction where you practice and what particular laws apply in that jurisdiction.

Although ideally, before entering practice, you will know the answer to every legal question that may arise over the course of your practice career, this of course is an unrealistic expectation. Therefore, you need an attorney on your team who is very familiar with the pertinent statutes and who can help answer questions as they arise in the course of day-to-day clinical practice. Many professional associations have a legal consultation plan in which a certain number of hours with an attorney may be purchased for an annual fee. This may serve as a valuable resource for the private practice clinician. There are also attorneys who specialize in mental health law and consultation to mental health practices. Contact your professional association and they will likely be able to identify such an attorney.

Attorneys should be asked to review important documents that you might be asked to sign in several aspects of your practice. This might include documents you are asked to sign in joining a group practice and contracts with managed care organizations (MCOs). Attorneys can also help you develop contracts for hiring an associate for the practice, creating a partnership, and hiring staff.

Although not specifically related to professional ethics, a CPA familiar with mental health practices will help ensure that you are properly following tax law. What is a tax-deductible expense and what is not is often not readily clear or can be open to interpretation. If a client fails to pay you the $35 on their balance due, can you deduct this as a business loss? Can you hire an associate as a 1099 independent contractor? If you attend a one-day professional meeting in another city, what costs of your three days away can be tax deductible? Is your consultation with the CPA deductible? It is important to understand the tax implications of the monies you are spending to run your practice. A CPA can also help you design a bookkeeping and record-keeping system that will help maintain appropriate and legal financial records. It is essential to have this in place as there is an ethical duty to communicate about financial issues with clients as part of the informed consent process.

To find a CPA familiar with mental health practices, we suggest polling colleagues regarding satisfaction with their current CPA. Ask those who are pleased with the service they are receiving if they would be willing to make a referral to that professional. It is essential that you feel comfortable working with your CPA so that you may make both sound business decisions and also decrease the likelihood you will make an ethical mistake. We have recently consulted with a private practitioner who felt intimidated by his CPA and therefore did not want to "appear stupid," so he limited his questions. As a result he did not fully understand the financials of his practice and thus ran the risk of making financial mistakes with clients. If you do not feel comfortable in working with your CPA (they actually should be working *for* you), we strongly suggest finding another CPA. Walfish and Barnett (2009) present an interview with Barry Melancom, president and CEO of the American Institute of Certified Public Accountants. In this interview he addresses important questions for mental health professionals as to why and when they should consult with CPAs, what services CPAs can provide to the mental health professional, and how to find an experienced CPA.

Walfish and Barnett (2009) point to the benefit of having "obsessive-compulsive tendencies" when billing and collecting for your practice. There are a tremendous number of details to follow in ensuring that you are practicing ethically. Barnett and Walfish (2011) spend an entire book examining ethics issues related to billing and collecting. Billing and collection procedures must be designed to protect each client's confidentiality. Take the frequent example of one member of a marital couple seeking counseling, but who does not want their spouse to know they have sought out the services of a counselor. How is the billing handled? If balances are due on the account, can you send a bill to the home and risk the spouse seeing an envelope with the return address "Jane Doe, LCPC"? If insurance is being used to help pay for the counseling, will an Explanation of Benefits be sent to the home, and will it in fact be sent to the spouse because the insurance is in his or her name? Does the employer (which provides the employee's insurance) get information as part of its utilization reports? These are but a few of the confidentiality issues involved in the billing and collecting process that the clinician must attend to in consultation with clients. Ethics issues related to billing and collecting are addressed in further detail in Chapter 5.

You are professionally responsible for your own billing and collecting, even if you have delegated this task to someone to complete on your behalf. It is difficult to know all of these details from the beginning. As such, until you have several years of experience under your belt, we think it essential to have a consultant available who can answer questions about these details. For example, we were recently with a psychologist new to practice. His client had been involved in a motor vehicle accident and was seeking services to help with the resulting anxiety. He wanted to use his regular employer-provided health insurance to pay for psychotherapy. However, the clinician was unaware that Box 10-B on the standard insurance claim form asks whether or not the client's condition is related to an auto accident. If he had not specifically checked the box indicating that it was related to an accident, he inadvertently would have been committing insurance fraud (in these instances the employer's health insurance carrier wants the auto insurance carrier to be responsible for the cost of psychotherapy). With this consultation the clinician avoided doing something illegal, even though there was no malice intended. Similarly, it is very important to be aware of your local laws regarding your obligations when you plan to pursue an unpaid bill from a patient. There are often many requirements incumbent on the professional.

With regard to other contracts, we recommend that a senior mental health professional review any contract that you might sign when considering joining a practice, hiring someone into your practice, or forming a partnership with other clinicians. The senior professional cannot offer legal advice, but can review the contract through the lens of what it will be like to provide professional services under the conditions of the contract. For example, such contract review can address what is mentioned about coverage provided in emergencies, or if the clinician is ill or on vacation. It can also address the ethics around noncompetition agreements and making sure clients have access to care when it is needed.

Walfish (2011) has written in an editorial that the ethics of noncompetition agreements should be called into question. An attorney can advise you on whether a noncompetition clause in a practice agreement fits the letter and spirit of the law in terms of limitations in geography (e.g., so many miles from the primary practice location) and time frame (how many years following the termination of the agreement). However, an attorney cannot advise you on the ethical impact of signing such an agreement that restricts the ability of a client to continue seeing you for psychotherapy once you leave the practice. Walfish (2011) has argued that if a restrictive covenant is in place and enforced, clients are the losers because they lose their autonomy and ability to choose to continue with the psychotherapist. Attorney Thomas Lewis describes in Walfish and Barnett (2009) the rationale of the New Jersey Supreme Court in banning noncompetition agreements for mental health professionals in that state, because the right of whom to see should lie with the client and not the mental health professional. It should be pointed out that this ruling does not extend beyond New Jersey, and to date no ethics committee that we know of has deemed it unacceptable to sign a noncompetition agreement.

At times, contractual issues may require the advice of all three consultants (i.e., an attorney, a CPA, and a senior mental health professional). For example, contractual agreements between a clinician and the practice they are joining often specify (a) the duties and responsibilities of the clinician and (b) the amount of administrative oversight the practice will have over the clinician's practice. At times it is clear that the clinician is being asked to join the practice as an independent contractor, whereas at other times it is clear that he or she is being asked to join as an employee. However, there certainly are situations where it becomes murky as to whether one is an employee or an independent contractor. The IRS has specific rules about this that focus on control of the person's behavior by the owner of the business. These rules can be explained and clarified by an attorney and CPA. However, it may take a senior-level clinician to understand how much autonomy the clinician actually has over their practice activities and patterns. For example, we have reviewed contracts in which a psychologist was asked to join a group practice. The contract specified that they needed to attend staff meetings on Monday mornings. Specific language was written into the contract that documentation and billing information needed to be completed on the day of service. There were many other stipulations in the contract that made it clear to us, as consultants reviewing the contract, that the clinician's work behavior was being controlled by the practice and thus they should have been viewed as an employee instead of as an independent contractor. This difference is not a semantic one, as both specifications have different legal and tax requirements for the employee and the practice.

LOCATION AND OFFICE SETTING

Mental health professionals have the flexibility to practice in a wide variety of settings. There is no prescription as to where you have to practice. For example, we have practices that were located in Class A Medical Office buildings, a town-house in a complex of professional offices that surrounded a duck pond, in houses that were refurbished into office space, and our own home. Each practice setting may bring certain challenges with them. As such, the mental health professional should take care to ensure the setting in which they practice meets contractual and ethical obligations to clients.

For example, physical accessibility to care is an important consideration in choosing where to practice. Many managed care contracts insist that, to be a pro-vider for that company, the office has to be handicapped accessible. This assures the carrier that their subscribers will not be discriminated against due to their disability. As such, the office where you practice must have hallways wide enough to accommodate a wheelchair, ramps that will allow the client to maneuver their wheelchair, and a suitable bathroom arrangement. These accommodations must be made to meet your contractual obligations. From a legal perspective, mental health professionals may need to comply with the accessibility requirements of the Americans with Disabilities Act (2002).

The ethics codes of each of the mental health professions all specify that pre-serving clients' confidentiality is paramount. Where you choose to practice may limit the clinician's ability to provide such assurance. For example, opening a prac-tice in a busy shopping mall may make sense from a visibility and business traf-fic perspective. However, if the store in the mall is called "Psychological Services Center," and everyone in the mall passing by can peek in the window and see who is waiting to see the psychologist, confidentiality is clearly compromised. That does not mean that you have to practice in an isolated setting. No client who visits a mental health professional is assured of 100% confidentiality. We have had the experience of clients meeting friends or associates in our waiting rooms. Clients may consider this an embarrassment.

This cannot be avoided, especially in small communities. However, sensitivity in scheduling clients is advised when you know there may be clients who know each other. For example, if you are seeing two employees who work at the same company, it may be best not to schedule them back to back. This decreases the likelihood that they will run into each other. Some offices are designed so clients enter a waiting room through one door, but exit through a separate door, thereby decreasing the likelihood that they will meet someone they know. Obviously this is not always prac-tical, but if you have the opportunity to design a space prior to build-out this should be considered. Similarly, in a multiclinician office there is no control over scheduling of another professional's clients. You obviously have no control over when another clinician schedules their clients, and one of your associates' clients may know one of your clients and may see each other in the waiting room. However, the probability of chance meetings between clients can easily be reduced by having more time between appointments in all practice settings, so later clients are not waiting when earlier ones are leaving, and by staggering start times of the clinicians in group practices, so that all clinicians don't start appointments at the top of the hour.

As mentioned, clinicians may have their practices in a variety of settings. Challenges to preserving confidentiality may exist in settings outside of a traditional private practice. For example, some universities allow faculty to use their offices in their Department of Psychology to see private-practice clients. Care must be taken to ensure these clients have privacy in these settings, just as if the service were being provided in a Class A Medical Office building. It must not be obvious that the person standing outside Dr. Smith's office is awaiting a psychotherapy appointment. Similarly, records must be stored in such a way that only Dr. Smith has access to them. Other settings that allow the use of an office in an institutional setting for private practice must also preserve the client's confidentiality.

What is discussed in the consulting room should be between the clients in the room and the clinician. It is distracting and distressing to clients to be (a) walking in the hall and able to hear conversations taking place in the other consulting rooms, and (b) sitting in their chair in the consulting room and being able to hear the client in the next room discussing the intimate details of their life. As such, although absolute soundproofing cannot be achieved, attempts to approximate soundproofing are essential in order to (a) preserve the confidentiality of the content being discussed in each clinician's office, and (b) provide an environment in which all clients feel safe to share intimate details of their lives and know they will be only heard by the people in the room.

Holohan and Slaikeu (1977) found that a reduced level of privacy decreases the amount of self-disclosure that may occur in counseling. In addition to adequate soundproofing, many clinicians use white noise machines or have music playing softly outside of their consultation room and in their waiting room. White noise machines can be purchased in office supply stores, and their use reduces the likelihood that private discussions will be heard by others outside of the room. If you are in the position of constructing office space, a useful strategy is to insulate inside the walls and ceilings and also to make sure the walls go all the way up (beyond the ceiling tiles) to the floor above (commonly referred to as the "deck").

Pressly and Heesacker (2011) present a review of the literature regarding the effects of the physical environment in which counseling takes place on the counseling process. According to these authors, it is important for counselors to decorate their offices in a way that is pleasing to them, as it is important for them to feel comfortable in their work environment. However, they also point out that "counselors should consider the potential effects of particular artwork on clients because research indicates that clients may differ in the interpretation of artwork.... may be perceived as sexually suggestive by some clients...and might offend the sensibilities of some clients" (p. 150).

So although the nude painting on the wall may be pleasing to the psychotherapist and artistically may be considered "a classic," the ethically informed clinician may choose not to place such a piece of artwork on their walls. Some may argue that the discomfort of the art is "grist for the therapeutic mill" to discuss with "a sexually repressed client," but it may also represent a lack of cultural sensitivity on the clinician's part.

ETHICAL CHALLENGES

- Licensing requirements vary by jurisdiction, including amount of postgraduate training needed and type of supervision that is acceptable to licensing boards.
- Clients rarely know the difference between someone who is licensed to practice independently and someone who is required to practice under supervision. This must be carefully explained to clients upon entering treatment.
- It is important to find a supervisor that will meet your specific needs for service delivery, practice development, and professional development.
- When in solo practice, especially as an early-career professional, it is difficult to know how to respond to the myriad of ethics issues and potential conflicts that arise in day-to-day practice. There are many days on which you will say to yourself, "We never discussed what to do when this happens when I was in graduate school."
- With the movement toward an increase in integrated health care practice, mental health professionals should be aware that they do not share the same ethics codes with these other health care providers.

KEY POINTS TO KEEP IN MIND

- Beginning a practice is logistically complex from a clinical and business standpoint, and there are important ethics issues that arise in all aspects of the development and maintenance of your practice.
- It is up to you to document work experience and supervision received. Keep careful records to ensure you are in compliance with what is required of you.
- Many supervisors have never received training in supervision. Therefore, it is important that you take an active role in shaping the supervision to ensure the experience meets your logistical and training needs.
- While practicing under supervision, you must not misrepresent your status as a professional in training, and you must never imply being an independently licensed professional.
- It takes a team of professionals (attorney, CPA, senior-level mental health clinician) to keep you informed of ethical and legal issues in both the clinical and business aspects of practice.
- When joining a practice of other professionals, they will want to know your ethical thought process. You should also know the ethical thought processes of the members of the group you are considering joining.
- Confidentiality is the hallmark of providing a safe environment for clients to discuss their problems and concerns. This should be one of

the paramount issues that guides all decisions regarding your practice behaviors.

- You are responsible for the behavior of support staff and those that interact with clients or outside parties on your behalf.
- Contracts that you are asked to sign are usually written in the best interest of those asking you to sign the contract. It is important that you understand the business, legal, and ethical implications of the wording included in the contract and that you advocate for the protection of your clients and business.

PRACTICAL RECOMMENDATIONS

- Be careful and compulsive in completing licensure applications.
- Have your "ethics team" in place prior to beginning your practice.
- If you are considering joining a group practice, interview with at least three of them before making a decision on which one to join.
- Become extremely knowledgeable of the licensing law in your jurisdiction as well as the ethics code of your profession.
- Have a supervision contract signed and in place prior to beginning the formal supervision relationship.
- Choose a supervisor that will not only teach you about clinical and business aspects of practice, but also whom you believe will be a role model for ethical practice.
- Have any contract that you sign reviewed by an attorney familiar with mental health practice as well as by a senior-level mental health professional.
- Make sure that all support staff are trained in maintaining client confidentiality and have a working agreement as to what constitutes appropriate professional behavior.
- Review the billing and collection procedures of a practice if they are performing this function on your behalf.
- Proactively, and on a continuous basis, have discussions related to ethics with other health care providers when practicing in their settings.

PITFALLS TO AVOID

- Do not practice in isolation.
- Do not be reluctant to spend money for professional consultation. It is an investment in your business.
- Do not be impulsive in choosing a practice arrangement, whether it be a solo practice or a group practice.
- Do not rely on "handshake agreements" regarding business or supervision agreements.

- Do not assume that support staff are sufficiently trained in issues related to confidentiality and professional behavior simply because they have been in the practice for a significant period of time.
- Do not "stick your head in the sand" about learning appropriate billing and collection procedures if they are delegated to someone who provides this service on your behalf.
- Do not bend your ethical obligations when practicing in alternative health care settings or feel that you have to defer to physicians regarding ethical decision making because you are practicing in their offices.

RELEVANT ETHICS CODE STANDARDS

Supervision

- American Association for Marriage and Family Therapy (AAMFT) Code of Ethics (AAMFT, 2012) Principle 4.5, Oversight of Supervisee Professionalism, states, "Marriage and family therapists take reasonable measures to ensure that services provided to supervisees are professional" (p. 3).
- American Counseling Association (ACA) Code of Ethics (ACA, 2005) Standard F.1.a., Client Welfare, states a "primary obligation of counseling supervisors is to monitor the services provided by other counselors or counselors-in-training. Counseling supervisors monitor client welfare and supervisee clinical performance and professional development" (p. 13).
- APA Ethics Code (APA, 2010) Standard 7.06, Assessing Student and Supervisee Performance, states, "(a) In academic and supervisory relationships, psychologists establish a timely and specific process for providing feedback to students and supervisees. Information regarding the process is provided to the student at the beginning of supervision. (b) Psychologists evaluate students and supervisees on the basis of their actual performance on relevant and established program requirements" (p. 10).
- National Association of Social Workers (NASW) Code of Ethics (NASW, 2008) Standard 3.01c, Supervision and Consultation, states, "Social workers should not engage in any dual or multiple relationships with supervisees in which there is a risk of exploitation or potential harm to the supervisee" (p. 9).

Scope of Practice

- AAMFT Code of Ethics (AAMFT, 2012) Principle 3.1 states, "Marriage and family therapists do not diagnose, treat, or advise on problems outside the recognized boundaries of their competence" (p. 2).

- ACA Code of Ethics (ACA, 2005) Standard C.2.d., Monitor Effectiveness, requires counselors to "continually monitor their effectiveness as professionals and take steps to improve when necessary" (p. 9).
- APA Ethics Code (APA, 2010) Standard 2.01a, Boundaries of Competence, states, "Psychologists provide services, teach and conduct research with populations and in areas within the boundaries of their competence, based on their education, training, supervised experience, consultation, study or professional experience" (p. 4).
- NASW Code of Ethics (2008) Standard 1.04 states: "Social workers should provide services and represent themselves as competent only within the boundaries of their education, training, and professional experience" (p. 6). Additionally, NASW Code of Ethics Standard 3.01 states: "Social workers who provide supervision or consultation should have the necessary knowledge and skill to supervise or consult appropriately and should do so only within their areas of knowledge and expertise" (p. 13).

Referrals and Renting Office Space

- AAMFT Code of Ethics (AAMFT, 2012) Principle 7.1, Financial Arrangements, states, "Marriage and family therapists do not offer or accept kickbacks, rebates, bonuses, or other remuneration for referrals" (p. 7).
- APA Ethics Code (APA, 2010) Standard 6.07, Referrals and Fees, states, "Payment is based on services provided...and is not based on the referral itself" (p. 9).

Office Space

- ACA Code of Ethics (ACA, 2005) Standard A.2.c., Developmental and Cultural Sensitivity, requires counselors to interact with clients and communicate with them in a manner that is respectful of clients' backgrounds and individual differences.
- APA Ethics Code (APA, 2010) Standard 2.01, Boundaries of Competence, states that when providing services to individuals of diverse backgrounds, "psychologists have or obtain the training, experience, consultation or supervision necessary to ensure the competence of their services" (p. 5).
- NASW Code of Ethics (NASW, 2008) Standard 4.02, Discrimination, states that social workers may not engage in any form of discrimination, including those based on mental or physical disabilities. Further, NASW Code of Ethics Standard 1.05, Cultural Competence and Social Diversity, requires that social workers have the knowledge and skills needed to effectively work with clients of varying backgrounds.

REFERENCES

American Association for Marriage and Family Therapy. (2012). *Code of ethics.* Retrieved from http://www.aamft.org/imis15/content/legal_ethics/code_of_ethics.aspx

American Counseling Association. (2005). *ACA code of ethics.* Retrieved from http://www.counseling.org/Resources/aca-code-of-ethics.pdf

American Psychological Association. (2010). *Ethical principles of psychologists and code of conduct.* Retrieved from http://www.apa.org/ethics

Americans With Disabilities Act. (2002). Retrieved from http://www.ada.gov/2010_regs.htm

Barnett, J. E. (2000). The supervisee's checklist: Ethical, legal, and clinical issues. *The Maryland Psychologist, 4,* 18–20.

Barnett, J. E. (2007). In search of the effective supervisor. *Professional Psychology: Research and Practice, 38,* 268–275.

Barnett, J. E. (2013, Summer). Clinical supervision basics and beyond. *Maryland Board of Examiners of Psychologists Newsletter,* 7–8, 10.

Barnett, J. E., & Walfish, S. (2011). *Billing and collecting for your mental health practice: Effective strategies and ethical practice.* Washington, DC: APA Books.

Bernard, J. M., & Goodyear, R. K. (2014). *Fundamentals of clinical supervision* (5th ed.). Upper Saddle River, NJ: Pearson Education.

Coons, H., & Gablis, J. (2010). Contractual issues for independent psychologists practicing in health care settings: Practical tips for establishing an agreement. *Independent Practitioner, 30,* 181–183.

Fisher, M. A. (2009). Ethics based training for nonclinical staff in mental health settings. *Professional Psychology: Research and Practice, 40,* 459–466.

Handelsman, M. M. (2001). Learning to become ethical. In S. Walfish & A. K. Hess (Eds.), *Succeeding in graduate school: The career guide for psychology students* (pp. 189–202). Mahwah, NJ: Erlbaum.

Health Insurance Portability and Accountability Act of 1996, Pub. L. 104-191, 110 Stat. 1936 (1996).

Holohan, C., & Slaikeu, K. (1977). Effects of contrasting degrees of privacy on client self-disclosure in a counseling setting. *Journal of Counseling Psychology, 24,* 55–59.

Hudgins, C., Rose, R., Fifield, P., & Arnault, S. (2013). Navigating the legal and ethical foundations of informed consent and confidentiality in integrated primary care. *Families, Systems, & Health, 31,* 9–19.

Kanzler, K. E., Goodie, J. L., Hunter, C. L., Glotfelter, M. A., & Bodart, J. J. (2013). From colleague to patient: Ethical challenges in integrated primary care. *Families, Systems, & Health, 31,* 41–48.

Kelly, J., & Coons, H. (2012). Integrated healthcare and professional psychology: Is the setting right for you? *Professional Psychology: Research and Practice, 43,* 586–595.

National Association of Social Workers. (2008). *Code of ethics.* Retrieved from http://www.socialworkers.org/pubs/code/code.asp

Nordal, K. (2012). Healthcare reform: Implications for independent practice. *Professional Psychology: Research and Practice, 43,* 535–44.

Pressly, P., & Heesacker, M. (2011). The physical environment and counseling: A review of theory and research. *Journal of Counseling and Development, 79,* 148–160.

Reiter, J., & Runyan, C. (2013). The ethics of complex relationships in primary care behavioral health. *Families, Systems, & Health, 31,* 20–27.

Runyan, C. (2011). Psychology can be indispensible to health care reform and the patient-centered medical home. *Psychological Services, 8*, 53–68.

Thomas, J. (2010). *The ethics of consultation and supervision: Practical guidance for mental health professionals.* Washington, DC: APA Books.

Walfish, S. (2011, Summer). Noncompetition clauses should be banned for psychologists. *Independent Practitioner, 31*, 139–140.

Walfish, S., & Barnett, J. E., (2009). *Financial success in mental health practice: Essential tools and strategies for practitioners.* Washington DC: APA Books.

Werth, J., Welfel, E., & Benjamin, G. A. (2008). *The duty to protect: Ethical, legal, and professional considerations for mental health professionals.* Washington DC: APA Books.

Woody, R. (2013). *Legal self-defense for mental health practitioners: Quality care and risk management strategies.* New York: Springer Books.

2

Clinical Practice

Entering into private practice represents the culmination of many years of hard work in graduate school, postlicensure work experience, and clinical supervision. Although private practice can be very rewarding personally and professionally, it also brings with it a number of ethical and legal challenges. Familiarity with these challenges and advanced planning can go a long way to assist you in preventing some of the difficulties we will describe in this chapter. Although it is assumed that all mental health professionals will endeavor to provide the best possible clinical care to their clients, failure to anticipate and prepare for these common challenges and dilemmas may prove deleterious for client and clinician alike.

SCOPE OF PRACTICE

Each mental health clinician will have to determine his or her scope of practice to ensure competent, ethical, and effective care for all clients served. One's *scope of practice* refers to the range of professional services and types of clients one may competently assess and treat. *Clinical competence* is generally thought to comprise "the habitual and judicious use of communication, knowledge, technical skills, clinical reasoning, emotions, values, and reflection in daily practice for the benefit of the individual and the community served" (Epstein & Hundert, 2002, p. 226). Additionally, clinical competence can be thought of as possessing the knowledge, skills, attitudes, and values needed to provide effective care and having the ability to implement them effectively (Barnett, Doll, Younggren, & Rubin, 2007).

Knowledge about working with clients is typically gained initially through academic coursework, whereas clinical skills are developed through supervised clinical experiences. Ethical values and behaviors are, one hopes, inculcated in every mental health professional throughout their training and through the course of their careers. The values of all mental health professions are articulated in their respective codes of ethics. Once in practice, clinicians may further develop their current competence, and even expand their scope of practice by establishing new areas of competence through additional education, training, and supervised clinical experience.

All mental health clinicians should consider their current clinical competence when deciding on the range of clients they will assess and treat, and the range of treatment techniques they will use. No mental health clinician will be competent in all areas of practice. There always will be types of clients (children, adolescents, adults, the elderly), diagnoses (anxiety disorders, depression, eating disorders, schizophrenia, abuse, addictions, etc.), treatment modalities (individual, group, couples, family), and techniques (psychotherapy, play therapy, hypnosis, biofeedback, EMDR, etc.) that require specific competencies and thus impact our ability to work with particular clients and meet their particular treatment needs.

In addition to being competent with regard to presenting problems, treatment techniques, and treatment modalities, it is vital that mental health clinicians keep in mind that presenting problems may have a range of meanings for individuals from different backgrounds. Clients' treatment needs may vary based on their individual differences; even how we interact and communicate with clients may need to be modified based on their individual differences and needs. Thus, it is an ethical imperative that all clinicians develop and maintain multicultural competence, so that we can provide clinical services effectively to all individuals who may seek our assistance (Erickson Cornish, Schreier, Nadkarni, Metzger, & Rodolfa, 2010). A careful ongoing analysis of the range and limits of our clinical and multicultural competence is essential to ensure that we meet each client's needs most appropriately and that we do not attempt to provide clinical services outside of our areas of competence.

Although self-awareness and self-assessment are essential steps for ensuring that we only practice within our scope of practice, these strategies have been shown to be quite limited in their effectiveness. A wide body of research demonstrates the general inaccuracy of—and in fact the typical overestimations of—our self-assessments of competence (Davis et al., 2006; Dunning, Heath, & Suls, 2004), and that the less competent we are, the more likely we are to self-assess inaccurately (Eva et al., 2004). Walfish, McAllister, O'Connell, and Lambert (2012) found that compared to their peers, 25% of mental health professionals rated their own skills to be at the 90th percentile or above, and none viewed themselves as being below average. Further, clinicians tended to overestimate rates of client improvement and underestimate rates of client deterioration (Dunning et al., 2004).

It is therefore important that we not serve as the sole judge of our own levels and limits of competence. Instead, we should work closely with trusted colleagues who can assist us with honest feedback. Further, when learning new skills under clinical supervision (or mentorship), we recommend that the determination of when the clinician is ready to begin using the new techniques or strategies be made independently, with the active input of one's clinical supervisor (or mentor). Each mental health clinician's scope of practice and limits of clinical competence will have a direct impact on how we market our professional services, which referrals we accept, and which we do not.

CLINICAL COMPETENCE AND ACCEPTING REFERRALS

As businesspeople, especially when first starting out in practice, we may be tempted to accept every referral that comes our way. Many pressures can influence our judgment about accepting referrals. These can include our financial obligations to our practice (rent, utilities, staff salaries, etc.) and in our personal lives (living expenses, student loans, saving for retirement, etc.). Mental health clinicians who are early in their careers may find it difficult to turn down referrals when they are focused on establishing or building one's practice. They may fear disappointing referral sources, fearing that they might not refer other clients in the future, in addition to turning away income when facing the aforementioned financial pressures.

With regard to financial pressures and the need to build one's practice, it is important to keep in mind our ethical obligations to those we serve. One can even consider the conflict between our financial needs and our clients' treatment needs to be a potential conflict of interest situation. To ensure ethical practice, we must weigh these competing demands so we do not place our own needs or motivations above our clients' clinical needs. Barnett and Walfish (2011) discuss countertransference issues that clinicians may face in the billing and collections process that have the potential for compromising ethical practice and procedures. Examples of such countertransference issues may include being phobic about possible client anger and allowing a large balance due to build up, being fearful of losing a client for economic reasons and thus avoiding difficult psychotherapeutic material, or routinely waiving copays so the client will appreciate this generous act. Although every mental health practitioner will want to have a busy and successful practice, we should endeavor to provide clients with the most competent and effective clinical services possible. Thus, thoughtful decisions need to be made about which clients to accept into one's practice and which referrals should be declined.

There is no exact standard to use or decision-making rubric to follow that will tell us what the best course of action is in each situation. Situations vary, but we may use ethical decision-making models, thoughtful consideration, and consultation with colleagues to make informed decisions. Although it is true that we need not be an expert in the area of practice relevant to each client's treatment needs, we must possess at least the minimum accepted level of competence to provide effective services. Practice guidelines promulgated by the various mental health professions are one source of information about minimally accepted standards, as are experienced colleagues who are recognized experts in the area of practice in question. When unsure, receiving clinical supervision or consultation from an expert colleague can be an important and helpful strategy. Seeking ongoing education and training can be helpful for enhancing and expanding clinical competence while treating a client or learning new assessment strategies or other practice service areas.

With regard to concerns about disappointing referral sources, it is helpful to keep in mind our goals in these situations. When a physician refers one of his or her patients, he or she is hoping to have that individual's mental health needs addressed in an effective manner. In essence, he or she wants the patient's problems taken care of effectively. This is not to suggest that the only way of achieving this goal is for you to accept the referral and to personally provide the treatment. Most referral sources will greatly appreciate it if you acknowledge the limits of your competence, while actively working to ensure that the patient's treatment needs are effectively met. Mental health clinicians can do this by assessing the client's treatment needs and then assisting the client to access the best services available to meet these needs. One can provide the client with the contact information of other colleagues who possess the needed competence, make contact with these colleagues to help expedite the referral process (with the client's consent), and then follow up with the client to ensure that they are receiving and are satisfied with needed services. If they are not, additional referrals can be made, again with active follow-up. Then, with the client's consent, the mental health clinician can report back to the referral source on actions taken and the reasons why this course was followed. Most referral sources will respect the clinician for recognizing and staying within their boundaries of competence, and will appreciate their efforts to meet their patient's treatment needs. Although the time involved in taking these actions is not billable, it may very likely be excellent customer service (Walfish & Barnett, 2009) that results in many future referrals from that individual. In fact, one of the authors found early in his career that not seeing a man who was chemically dependent, but instead recommending to the referring physician a local treatment facility where the patient could be immediately evaluated, was instrumental in building an excellent long-standing referral partnership. The physician viewed the "refusal" of the referral as an act of patient-centered integrity.

Another option is to accept the referral on a conditional basis. This can occur by specifically stating to the patient and the referral source (if appropriate) that the first few visits will be a "consultation," during which you will assess the patient's needs, treatment options, and the fit and appropriateness of working together. This can be especially important when seeing cases about which you may have some uncertainty regarding the ultimate appropriateness of the referral. For example, although you might be comfortable having some patients in acute crisis in your caseload with a personality disorder, you might find that having more than two or three of these patients at one time is overwhelming and can diminish your effectiveness. Having a two-stage intake process (the consultation and then treatment, rather than just beginning with treatment) can help ensure you do not find yourself inundated with cases that go beyond your abilities or stress tolerance level. It can also provide you with the ability to make a more targeted referral of the patient so ideally they can receive optimal care going forward.

WAIT TIME AND WAITING LISTS

In addition to clinical competence, waiting time until the first appointment is available can be a relevant factor to consider when deciding whether to accept a referral. Although of course every mental health clinician will be pleased to have a practice that is so busy that potential clients are placed on a waiting list, such placement may not be appropriate for every client.

Thus, an initial brief screening of each client's treatment needs via telephone, when first contacted, will have two objectives. As described earlier, mental health clinicians must first determine if they possess the needed clinical competence to meet the client's treatment needs. If this competence is determined to be present, the level of urgency of the client's treatment needs must be considered. Some clients will be quite pleased to be placed on a waiting list and will feel some sense of relief to know that they have successfully made initial contact with the clinician and that they soon may be receiving treatment. Additionally, one can give the client an appointment in the future with the understanding that he or she will be contacted if an appointment opens up sooner.

Other clients, especially those in crisis or who are seeking emergency services, will not be suitable for placement on a waiting list. Thus, the clinician should consider the urgency of each client's treatment needs when considering placing prospective clients on a waiting list. This process may begin appropriately even before the initial appointment or intake interview. A good practice is to briefly assess the urgency of the client's presenting problems over the telephone when he or she makes initial contact. For those who are in crisis or who need emergency services, assistance can be provided such as scheduling a meeting immediately, if appropriate, or if not, recommending that they call 911 or go to the nearest emergency room. For those clients who can reasonably wait until the next available appointment time, placement on a waiting list may be appropriate. Clients who cannot wait due to some level of clinical urgency can be referred to colleagues who possess the needed competence and can meet the necessary urgency.

We recommend that clients placed on waiting lists be provided with the opportunity for informed consent (even at this stage) so that they will have realistic expectations about the amount of time they may remain in this status. The informed consent should address the clinician's brief assessment of the client's clinical status, possible risks and signs of exacerbation, and what steps the client should take if their clinical condition becomes more acute. In essence, each party's obligations and expectations of the other should be discussed and agreed upon from the outset.

UNDERSTANDING INFORMED CONSENT

Informed consent is an interactive process between clinician and client that begins at the outset of the professional relationship and continues through its ending (Fisher & Oransky, 2008). Informed consent involves sharing a sufficient amount of information with the client so that he or she may make an educated decision about participation in the services being offered. The mental health professions'

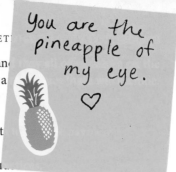

codes of ethics all require that this process occur, an
issues that should be included in this discussion. At a

- A description of the services to be offered.
- Likely fees and relevant financial arrangement
  policies, the use of insurance, and the like.
- Frequency of appointments and scheduling p
- Confidentiality and its limits.
- Possible risks and benefits of treatment.
- Reasonably available alternatives and their likely risks and benefits (to
  include not participating in treatment).
- What to do should an emergency arise, as well as how and when to contact
  the clinician in between treatment sessions.

It is required that the informed consent process for treatment be conducted verbally and in writing (a written agreement signed by the client), that the client
is competent to give consent (cognitively and emotionally, as well as legally),
that clinicians actively ensure the client's understanding of what they are agreeing to, and that consent is given voluntarily (Barnett, Wise, Johnson-Greene, &
Buckey, 2007). Informed consent should be considered an ongoing process, not a
one-time event. As such, it should be updated whenever significant changes to the
agreed-upon treatment plan are anticipated.

When deciding on what information to share in the informed consent process
and in how much detail, legal requirements should be considered. Thus, mental health clinicians should carefully review their profession's code of ethics and
relevant licensing laws for these requirements. Additionally, goals of informed
consent should be considered to include the promotion of the treatment alliance
and a collaborative working relationship, lessening of the risk of exploitation and
reduction of the imbalance of power in the relationship, and the promotion of
the client's autonomous functioning (Younggren, Fisher, Foote, & Hjelt, 2011).
Consideration of these goals of informed consent should be helpful in determining how best to implement this process.

ASSENT

It is important that professional services only be provided to those individuals who have the legal right to consent to their own treatment, or for whom the
appropriate individual(s) provides consent on the other person's behalf. In most
jurisdictions a minor (typically an individual under 18 years of age) does not have
the legal right to consent to their own treatment. Because jurisdictions vary on
this, however, mental health clinicians should consult the relevant laws in their
own jurisdiction. For example, in Maryland, a minor of 16 or 17 years of age may
consent to their own treatment with a licensed psychologist, a licensed physician,
or at a hospital or clinic (State of Maryland, Family Law Article).

When minors do not possess the legal right to consent to their own treatment, a parent or guardian will typically provide this for them. It is essential that the clinician clarify from the outset which parent actually has this right. In cases of divorce it may not be readily apparent who possesses this legal right. It is important to ascertain this information at the intake interview and then only to provide additional professional services after receiving appropriate consent. In the case of an intact family, either parent may independently consent to their minor child's treatment. However, the parents in an "intact" family may be in disagreement about whether or not they want the child to be in treatment. When there is a great deal of conflict between the parents, it is often advisable to get consent from both parents before beginning treatment to avoid a situation where one parent permits you see the child, and the other parent then calls you to discontinue care. Although technically only one parent's consent is needed in such an intact-family situation, the prudent clinician may choose to proceed only with both parents' consent due to the significant level of conflict that might otherwise be present, which could limit one's ability to provide effective treatment.

When child custody has been contested, there will be a court order that specifies which parent retains this legal right, and thus whose consent is needed (one of the parents', or both). In these situations it is best to obtain a copy of the court order for your records prior to providing any additional services to the minor client, to ensure that you completely understand the order and that no individual's legal rights are violated or misrepresented. There are also times when a grandparent or another individual is actually the guardian and holds the legal right to authorize treatment. The court order may specify that one parent has final say over medical decision making for the minor child. However, it must be clarified whether mental health treatment falls under the category of medical treatment, otherwise one of the parents may claim that "counseling" is not medical in nature and therefore the other parent does not have decision-making authority.

Although minors typically are not legally authorized to provide their own informed consent to treatment, as a matter of effective clinical practice it is advisable to include the minor client in the information-sharing and decision-making process, a process called *assent*. Depending on the minor client's age, developmental level, maturity, and intellectual sophistication, decisions will be made on how much information to share with the minor client, at what level it will be shared, and how much he or she will actually participate in the decision-making process (Kuther, 2003). Clarifying the expectations of the minor client and the parent(s) or guardian(s) from the outset is consistent with the goals of informed consent reviewed earlier and should contribute to the likelihood of achieving desired clinical outcomes.

The informed consent and assent processes provide an important opportunity to clarify expectations of all involved. When providing clinical services to minors, several key issues will be relevant in this decision-making process. The issue of confidentiality will always be important to address and an agreement of all parties will be needed before treatment may begin. The parent or guardian who authorizes the treatment will typically have the legal right of access to all that transpires in treatment (though this varies by jurisdiction) and all that the minor client shares. However, enforcing this right will likely interfere with the development of a trusting relationship between the minor client and the clinician and may result in the client refusing to share information necessary for making optimal gains in treatment, or even to participate in treatment. Of course, differences will exist among clients, especially based on age and developmental level, but these expectations will need to be negotiated and agreed to at the beginning of the professional relationship (Koocher, 2007). For example, it will be important for the mental health clinician to help the parent of an adolescent client understand the need for a certain degree of confidentiality in the treatment process. Confidentiality will never be absolute, however, based both on legal requirements and clinical need, so agreement will need to be reached up front about what types of information will be kept confidential and addressed in treatment and what will be disclosed to the parent(s) or guardian(s). Because it is not possible to develop an exhaustive list of all possible circumstances, reasonably anticipated examples can be provided (e.g., the presence of suicidality or engaging in high-risk behaviors such as substance abuse, unprotected sex, or self-mutilation, among others) and the clinician's decision-making process for making these decisions can be shared (Koocher, 2007). This will help ensure that the minor client and parent(s) alike make informed decisions about the proposed course of treatment and their participation in it.

EXCEPTIONS TO CONFIDENTIALITY

As just mentioned, absolute confidentiality in the psychotherapy relationship does not exist. Instead, relative confidentiality is what can be expected, as should be specified in the informed consent agreement (Barnett et al., 2007). A number of limits to confidentiality exist, such as the parent(s)' or guardian(s)' right to access to treatment information, disclosures to insurance companies (with permission from the client) to receive coverage for clinical services provided, and when treatment is court-ordered, among others. Mandatory exceptions to confidentiality also exist and are specified in relevant statutes. Because variations exist among these laws, mental health clinicians are advised to become familiar with the specifics of these laws in their jurisdiction so that they can make sure their clients are fully informed as well.

Mandatory Reporting Requirements

Each jurisdiction has laws relevant to the reporting of a reasonable suspicion of abuse or neglect of minors. Although the specific wording of the law in each jurisdiction is of great importance, each specifies the standards for this required exception to confidentiality. Most of these laws pertain to a mental health professional having a reasonable suspicion, not definitive proof, of the occurrence of physical or sexual abuse, or neglect, that the professional has learned of in the context of his or her professional role. These laws provide standards for determining this reasonable suspicion, definitions of abuse and neglect to be considered, and specific reporting requirements that address when the report must be made and to whom. Note also that the professional is not required to actually perform an investigation. That is left up to the investigatory agency.

Most jurisdictions also have mandatory reporting requirements that address elder abuse and neglect or, in some jurisdictions, more broadly defined vulnerable-adult reporting requirements. Similar to minors, who rely on others for their day-to-day safety and welfare, adults in a similar status are also considered to be part of a vulnerable population and thus entitled to protection by the jurisdiction. *Vulnerable adults* may include elderly individuals who do not live independently and who are dependent on others for their well-being and care, but others, such as disabled adults of any age, may fall into this protected category as well. Often, these laws address abuse, neglect, exploitation, and self-neglect of these individuals.

It should also be pointed out that although mandatory reporting laws are in place in most jurisdictions, at times mental health clinicians have been known to choose to ignore these responsibilities (Brossig & Kalichman, 1992; Kalichman & Craig, 1991). Legal requirements, clinician characteristics, and situational dimensions have been found to interact in ways that influence child abuse reporting decisions. Mental health clinicians should be mindful of such factors and remain cognizant of their legal, ethical, and moral obligations in these situations. Additionally, one should not expect that a claim of ignorance will suffice as a legal explanation.

Dangerousness and Exceptions to Confidentiality

An additional required exception to confidentiality pertains to dangerousness situations based on the landmark *Tarasoff* case (1974/1976). Laws based on the ruling of this case pertain to the threat to do harm, to an identifiable victim or group of victims, made by a client to the mental health professional. Laws vary on the specifics of the clinician's obligations when a client shares such a threat, but these laws pertain to a duty to warn, a duty to protect, and/or a duty to treat. Knowing which of these are allowed and/or required in one's jurisdiction is essential for ensuring appropriate action in these situations. The importance of knowing these laws is underscored by data reported by Werth, Welfel, and Benjamin (2008), who found that 75% of clinicians surveyed were misinformed about their duties when working with a client that was potentially dangerous.

The duty to warn involves making a reasonable good-faith effort to contact and warn the intended victim of the imminent threat. The duty to protect pertains to contacting the police or other most appropriate entity or person and notifying them of the specifics of the threat so that they may take actions to protect the intended victim. The duty to treat, which is allowed in some jurisdictions, provides the mental health clinician the option of addressing the client's danger-ousness in treatment as long as doing so removes the imminent risk of harm to the intended victim, such as involuntary commitment of the client, thus removing the need to take actions to warn and protect.

This final point is of direct relevance to the concept of duty of care (Shapiro & Smith, 2011). Clinicians should keep in mind their obligation to their clients to provide the most appropriate care possible, even when dangerousness situa-tions arise. Thus, breaching confidentiality through warning the intended victim and notifying the authorities of the threat to do harm are not the only options available to clinicians. When consistent with the laws of one's jurisdiction, actions such as increasing the frequency or intensity of treatment, referral for medication consultation, the inclusion of family members or other members of the client's support system in treatment, and even voluntary commitment, may be appropri-ate means of fulfilling our mutual obligations to care for our clients and to protect others from harm.

In addition to being familiar with the relevant laws and regulations in one's jurisdiction that affect confidentiality, it is important that each exception to con-fidentiality be addressed as part of the informed consent process. This is essential, as each client has the right to decide what information they want to share with their psychotherapist based on their accurate understanding of how that informa-tion will be used, and the extent of the protections of their confidentiality they can anticipate.

A related issue is that of dangerousness to oneself. Each mental health clinician should assess every new client for the presence of suicidal ideation, intent, and plans. As with other forms of dangerousness, when voluntary outpatient treat-ment is possible it should be the first-choice intervention. But, there may be times when a client's suicidal risk is so great, that family members or significant others may need to be included in treatment, or involuntary inpatient treatment may be necessary. In anticipation of such possibilities, it is essential that mental health clinicians address these potential exceptions to confidentiality in the informed consent process (Jobes, Overholser, Rudd, & Joiner, 2008).

BOUNDARIES AND MULTIPLE RELATIONSHIPS

Boundaries

Boundaries are described as the ground rules of the professional relationship (Gutheil & Gabbard, 1993). They provide structure, clarify expectations, and set standards for appropriate interactions with clients. Boundaries include factors such as touch, self-disclosure, interpersonal space, location, and the giving and receiving of gifts. Boundaries may be avoided, crossed, or violated. With regard to the boundary of touch, for example, avoiding this boundary would include hav-ing a no-touching rule for treatment staff working with inpatients in treatment for sexual abuse. Although of course all boundaries do not need to be avoided, such as the boundary crossing of shaking a client's hand upon meeting for the first time, in some circumstances this is the most clinically appropriate course of action.

A *boundary crossing* is an action regarding one of these boundaries that is clinically relevant and appropriate. It is consistent with the client's history and treatment needs, and consistent with applicable ethics standards and laws. It is not unwelcomed by the client, and not motivated by the mental health clinician's personal needs, but instead by the client's treatment needs (Smith & Fitzpatrick, 1995). In contrast, a *boundary violation* conflicts with any of these criteria, and by definition, is seen as harmful, exploitative, and unethical (Younggren & Gottlieb, 2004).

Some flexibility exists about what determines the difference between a boundary crossing and a boundary violation. For example, cultural and other diversity factors may have a significant impact on what a client defines as a welcomed boundary crossing or an intrusive and inappropriate boundary violation. Similarly, the client's personal and mental health history may result in what a clinician intends as a helpful boundary crossing being perceived by the client as an intrusive and inappropriate boundary violation (e.g., when a client who had been abused cowered in response to the clinician offering a "high five" following a particularly impressive accomplishment of the client). Last, individual factors for the mental health clinician may determine if an action is a boundary crossing or violation. Examples include one's theoretical orientation and the intent of one's actions. For example, client-centered psychotherapists often are more comfortable with self-disclosure and the use of touch than psychoanalytic or psychodynamic psychotherapists, who are likely to be more conservative in their approach to boundaries in clinical practice. Actions motivated by one's personal needs and interests, rather than the client's treatment needs and best interests, will likely be seen as inappropriate boundary violations. For example, spending extra time with an attractive client because one finds the client so interesting to speak with is quite different from allowing a session to run over the allotted time due to the client being in crisis.

Although some care must be taken in deciding which actions are appropriate and likely to be considered boundary crossings, rigidly avoiding all boundaries in an attempt to avoid violations is not recommended. Overly rigid boundaries and a refusal to engage in appropriate boundary crossings that are consistent with the client's treatment needs may actually result in harm to the treatment relationship and undermine treatment effectiveness. Thus, refusing ever to engage in self-disclosure when its appropriate use might be a powerful and meaningful intervention for a client, or refusing ever to touch a client (e.g., a gentle touch on the forearm of a grieving client), might do more harm than good. When unsure about the use of boundary crossings, we recommend that mental health clinicians consult with experienced colleagues and utilize the educative functions of ethics committees. Further, when unsure about how a client will perceive or react to a planned action, it is best to openly discuss the planned action with the client first.

Multiple Relationships

Multiple relationships pertains to engaging in additional relationships with a client, or a significant other in a client's life, in addition to the primary professional relationship (Smith & Fitzpatrick, 1995). A range of possible multiple relationships exist, including personal or social relationships, business relationships, and romantic or sexually intimate relationships, among others. Although not all multiple relationships with clients are necessarily inappropriate, those that hold a significant risk of exploitation and harm of the client, and those that can reasonably be expected to adversely impact the clinician's objectivity and judgment, should be avoided.

A number of factors should be considered when contemplating entering into a multiple relationship with a client. Each mental health profession's code of ethics and licensing laws provide guidance on the parameters of appropriate and inappropriate multiple relationships. Although all inappropriate multiple relationships should be avoided because of the harm they can bring to clients, some care must be used in deciding on the appropriateness of multiple relationships, and for those that are entered, some care in managing them is needed.

Historically it has been shown that mental health professionals who engaged in inappropriate sexual intimacies with their patients had engaged in a series of increasingly intrusive boundary crossings and violations that preceded the sexual relations (Gutheil & Gabbard, 1993). This is termed *the slippery slope*. Because it was believed that all sexual intimacies were preceded by such an increasingly intrusive pattern, it was therefore concluded that all boundary crossings constitute being on the slippery slope and, as a result, will lead to harmful boundary violations and inappropriate multiple relationships.

In fact, it has been shown that this is not necessarily the case (Gottlieb & Younggren, 2009). Indeed, a mental health clinician may engage in appropriate and clinically indicated boundary crossing (e.g., acknowledging a personal history of infertility when providing psychotherapy for individuals or couples coping with infertility) without this leading to boundary violations. Further, one may even engage in appropriate and clinically indicated multiple relationships (e.g., regularly going to the same church as the client) without harming the client. In fact, there are times when a refusal to engage in an appropriate multiple relationship with a client may be what is harmful, because the client is then prohibited from accessing needed clinical services (Zur, 2007).

In rural (Firestone & Barnett, 2012) and other small, isolated, or closed environments, multiple relationships are a way of life (Schank, Helbok, Haldeman, & Gallardo, 2010). In such settings where one both lives and works, mental health professionals provide clinical services to the members of their community with whom they interact in varying roles and capacities on a daily basis. Although not all multiple relationships in these settings will be considered appropriate, a refusal to engage in any multiple relationships would remove the possibility of treating any member of the community.

One special form of a multiple relationship exists when, as a clinician, you serve more than one professional role with the same client(s). This can occur, for example, when you provide both psychotherapy and psychological testing, or when you see an adult for individual work and then simultaneously or sequentially provide couple counseling, or when you provide divorce mediation to parents and also serve as their child's psychotherapist. Here as with the other examples mentioned, the risks and benefits of the multiple relationships should be carefully assessed in advance of providing the service. A general guideline is to take great care before serving in these multiple roles so as to avoid the pitfalls that can affect the patient(s) by the possibility of there being an actual or perceived bias in your professional judgment.

How the mental health clinician manages boundaries and multiple relationships is of great importance. It is important to address boundary expectations as part of the informed consent process and to thoughtfully consider whether a preexisting multiple relationship precludes a viable treatment relationship due to impaired objectivity and judgment, or due to the presence of a significant risk of exploitation to or harm of the client. For example, in a rural setting a mental health clinician might need to provide treatment services to the child of a neighbor if there is no other appropriately trained mental health professional available. Yet, providing treatment to the spouse of one's employer might prove too great a risk for impaired objectivity and judgment.

In addition to consultation with expert colleagues and ethics committees, the use of an ethical decision-making model when faced with these dilemmas is strongly recommended. One general decision-making model provided by Barnett and Johnson (2009) may help guide mental health professionals to logically think through the various factors relevant to their decision making. There is much more detail to the model, but the basic steps involved include:

Stage 1: Define the Situation Clearly.
Stage 2: Determine Who Will Be Affected.
Stage 3: Refer to Both Underlying Ethical Principles and the Standards of [your profession's] Code of Ethics.
Stage 4: Refer to Relevant Laws/Regulations and Professional Guidelines.
Stage 5: Reflect Honestly on Personal Feelings and Competence.
Stage 6: Consult With Trusted Colleagues.
Stage 7: Formulate Alternative Courses of Action.
Stage 8: Consider Possible Outcomes for All Parties Involved.
Stage 9: Make a Decision and Monitor the Outcome. (pp. 143–145)

With regard to the situation of entering into a sexual or romantic multiple relationship with a former client, Younggren and Gottlieb's (2004) decision-making model provides the following specific questions mental health professionals may ask themselves to guide them in this decision-making process:

1. Is this multiple relationship necessary or avoidable?
2. Can this type of relationship be a potential harm for the client?

3. Is there potential for the relationship to be beneficial?
4. Can I evaluate it objectively? (p. 267)

Honestly answering these questions can help guide mental health clinicians in their decision-making process when considering entering into multiple relationships so that clients' best interests are upheld.

When a multiple relationship is not contraindicated and avoiding it might do more harm than good (such as refusing treatment to an individual in great need when the risk or harm is slight and no other treatment resources exist in the local area), a helpful strategy is to compartmentalize the two relationships (Barnett & Yutrenzka, 1994). As would be agreed to in the informed consent process, the mental health clinician and client would compartmentalize the two relationships. When meeting for treatment sessions, only treatment issues will be discussed and that time will not be used to address issues from the other relationship. When interacting in the other relationship (e.g., customer at a client's store, serving on a civic committee together), only issues relevant to this other relationship will be discussed and clinical issues will not be addressed, saving them to be addressed in the treatment relationship.

ADDITIONAL BOUNDARY AND MULTIPLE RELATIONSHIP CHALLENGES

A number of boundary and multiple relationship challenges may arise during the course of mental health practice. For example, a client may offer their psychotherapist a gift. The professional literature typically draws a distinction between a gift valued at under $10 and those that are valued at more than this (Brown & Trangsrud, 2008). As with other boundary issues, we recommend a thoughtful decision-making process. Mental health clinicians should consider, for example, the client's age, the nature of the ongoing professional relationship, the potential meaning of the gift to the client and to the professional, any cultural or other diversity factors that may be relevant, and the clinician's theoretical orientation (e.g., whether it is "grist for the mill," or a simple "thank you" is the best response). Considering these factors can assist the mental health clinician in making an appropriate decision. For example, to accept a plate of baked goods from a psychotherapy client in December at holiday time would be seen as very different in meaning, intent, and impact on the clinician than accepting a gift of an expensive piece of jewelry from a wealthy client who is participating in a contested divorce and custody evaluation (Vasquez, 2007).

A second dilemma that may arise is being invited to attend a client's life event, such as a high school graduation, wedding, or birthday celebration. Although it is possible that the client simply wants to share this important milestone with their psychotherapist, an individual they may view as very important in their life, these are situations that raise a number of issues and challenges. First and foremost, this is a clinical issue that should be openly discussed during treatment sessions. The client's motivations and the meaning of having their psychotherapist attend the event should be considered.

When considering attending such an event, it is important to openly discuss issues such as how the client anticipates the event unfolding, what the psychotherapist's potential role or participation will be, how client confidentiality will be affected, and any potential implications for the ongoing professional relationship. As with all boundary and multiple relationships issues there may be times when attending such an event may be consistent with treatment needs, the treatment relationship, and the client's best interests. For example, a mental health clinician may be invited to the high school graduation of a client who had previously dropped out of high school, and only through the ongoing work in treatment with the clinician was he or she able to arrive at this important and momentous occasion. The mental health clinician may decide to attend the graduation ceremony, but also might decide not to attend the party with family and friends afterwards, in consideration of the boundary issues mentioned earlier. In all these situations the use of consultation, an ethical decision-making process, open discussion with the client, and consideration of the potential impact on the client of taking or not taking the intended action, should all occur before the clinician acts.

EMERGENCIES AND CRISES

As part of the informed consent process, it is important to include discussion of agreed-upon procedures for crises and emergencies. Doing so helps clients to know when to contact the professional in between appointments and how to do so. It is also vital that mental health professionals provide clients with easy access to themselves, or another designated colleague or care center if they are unavailable, so that clients' crises and emergencies are addressed in a timely manner.

This obligation does not require clinicians to be personally accessible to their clients 24 hours each day and seven days each week (something that would be contradictory to the requirement to practice appropriate self-care and wellness promotion needed to ensure clinical competence). Rather, we must make arrangements for appropriate emergency coverage. This can include the use of a group of colleagues who provide coverage for one another on a rotating basis. Of course, the nature of one's practice will influence the steps taken in this regard. Those with a small practice with few emergencies may find that providing clients with their cell phone number and instructions on when to use it may suffice.

When a mental health professional will be away from the office for an extended period of time, we suggest that calling in to check on one's voicemail messages is not a good practice for handling emergency situations. Instead, we recommend using colleagues to provide coverage in one's absence. However, it is best if clients are first informed of these coverage arrangements. For those clients whose crises may be anticipated, we suggest that a colleague who has the clinical competence and expertise specifically needed to assist that client be selected to provide coverage. It also may prove helpful, with the client's consent, to provide this colleague with information about the client's history, difficulties, and treatment, to possibly include providing this colleague with access to the client's treatment record.

Failure to make such arrangements is not consistent with prevailing professional practice standards and violates standards in the codes of ethics of the mental health professions. In fact, failure to be reasonably accessible to clients in between treatment sessions and during periods away from the office, or to make alternative arrangements to address the clients' ongoing treatment needs, may constitute abandonment of the client (Younggren et al., 2011). A key point here is to ensure that the needs of the clients are addressed. This is of course dependent on the clinical presentation, severity, and needs of the client(s). So, as mentioned, it is important to do what is clinically appropriate and reasonable based on the type of practice and clinical presentation of one's patient(s).

It is also important to address these issues in the informed consent agreement so that clients will have realistic expectations of their psychotherapist and will understand agreed-upon emergency procedures. In a life-or-death emergency situation it may not be appropriate to contact the mental health clinician. In these situations, going immediately to one's local emergency room or calling 911 may be the most prudent course of action. Each of these scenarios should be discussed and agreed to during the informed consent process so that emergencies and crises are responded to in the most appropriate way possible should they arise.

Mental health professionals must also plan for unanticipated absences such as illness, disability, and even death. Although these may be unpleasant and uncomfortable to consider, we must keep in mind our obligations to our clients and the need to take necessary precautions so their ongoing clinical needs will be addressed. Clinicians in a group practice may work out an arrangement with other group members to provide emergency coverage for them and to step in and address client needs should the clinician become unavailable to continue in practice. Solo practitioners maintain the same obligations but may find it more challenging to fulfill them. One important recommendation is to create a professional will (Bradley, Hendricks, & Kabell, 2012). This document specifies a colleague who has agreed to step in if the mental health professional is incapacitated or otherwise unable to continue in practice. This colleague is granted access to client records and contact information; thus clients should be informed of this as part of their informed consent agreement. This colleague contacts the clinician's clients upon learning of the unfortunate situation, explains the situation to the clients, meets with those clients who are in crisis or distress, and assists each client through the referral process to ensure that their ongoing treatment needs are met. This colleague is compensated for the time involved in carrying out these duties as agreed upon in advance and specified in the professional will, to be paid by the incapacitated clinician's estate.

TERMINATION AND ABANDONMENT

Termination is the ending of the professional relationship. Discussion of termination practices, policies, procedures, and expectations should begin as part of the informed consent process so that clients have realistic expectations about the course of treatment and its ending. There are a number of ways that the professional relationship may end. The most desired ending is the achievement of the agreed-upon goals of treatment. Clients may also leave treatment due to dissatisfaction with their progress or loss of interest in continued treatment, because they move their residence from the local area, or as a result of exhausting their insurance benefits or otherwise no longer being able to afford treatment. Mental health professionals may decide to end their work with a client due to the client's failure to comply with treatment recommendations, inconsistency in attending scheduled treatment sessions, failure to make progress in treatment or signs that the client is being harmed by treatment, the professional not possessing the necessary competence to meet the client's treatment needs, the discovery or development of an inappropriate multiple relationship, or the client not meeting the agreed-upon financial arrangements to pay for professional services rendered.

Regardless of the reason for ending the professional relationship, it is important that the mental health professional address the client's ongoing treatment needs. If such needs exist and the client will not, cannot, or should not continue in treatment with this professional, then appropriate referrals should be made. Although mental health professionals are under no obligation to treat clients indefinitely, we must make a reasonable good-faith effort to ensure that clients' ongoing treatment needs will be addressed (Younggren et al., 2011). For those clients we cannot continue treating who are in need of ongoing treatment, making referrals is required so that we are making a good-faith effort to ensure continuity of care. In those situations when a client misses appointments, or withdraws from or discontinues treatment, and our professional judgment indicates the need for ongoing treatment, we recommend contacting the client (typically best done in writing by letter) to make the recommendation for ongoing treatment, either with ourselves or, if desired, with colleagues to whom we can refer the client (Vasquez, Bingham, & Barnett, 2008). For an example, see the sample letter at the end of this chapter.

ETHICAL CHALLENGES

- Knowing the boundaries of your clinical competence and when not to accept referrals can be challenging. Relying on your own self-assessment in these situations can be especially problematic.
- Caution should be used in placing clients on waiting lists. Ensure the appropriateness of doing so and provide clients with informed consent about their status and actions to take should their condition change.
- Referral sources may desire feedback on the patients they refer to you. Be sure this is addressed in the informed consent process and that you act in compliance with your patient's wishes and best interests.
- Ensuring that informed consent is provided effectively can be challenging. Relying on clients signing written documents alone should be viewed as insufficient for achieving valid consent.

- Balancing the rights and needs of parents and their minor children who are our clients can be especially challenging. Thoughtfully addressing these expectations and plans in the informed consent process is essential.
- At times, clients' clinical needs and our legal obligations may come into conflict. Consultation with colleagues and legal professionals, and the use of a decision-making model, can be especially helpful in these situations.
- Determining which actions are boundary crossings and which ones are boundary violations can be very challenging, and there are a number of factors to be considered in making this determination.
- Determining when entering into multiple relationships is acceptable or necessary and when they should be avoided can be quite confusing, especially in small communities where limited options and alternatives exist.
- We must make arrangements for accessibility and addressing crises in between sessions and during periods of absence that are adequately responsive to our clients' ongoing needs.
- Ending the professional relationship must be done in a manner that addresses any ongoing clinical needs a client may have, to ensure that clients are not abandoned.

KEY POINTS TO KEEP IN MIND

- Always practice within your scope of practice and use caution when accepting referrals of clients whose clinical needs may exceed your clinical competence.
- Consult professional practice guidelines and experienced colleagues when unsure of the competencies needed to effectively provide particular services.
- Carefully monitor your clinical competence and take needed steps to maintain competence and to enhance or expand it when needed.
- Attend to self-care and the promotion of wellness, monitoring the effects of ongoing stressors that may adversely impact professional functioning.
- When accepting referrals, carefully consider each client's individual situation. Only place a prospective client on a waiting list if it is clinically appropriate to do so. If not, assist the client with appropriate referrals.
- Utilize a comprehensive informed consent process with each client at the outset of professional services, updating it as is needed throughout the course of the professional relationship.
- For those clients unable to provide their own consent to treatment, explain the services to be provided in a manner the client is most likely to understand and obtain consent from a legally appropriate third party.
- Address each party's expectations to include confidentiality and reach an agreement that is in the client's best interests prior to initiating treatment.

- Be knowledgeable of all legal exceptions to confidentiality in your jurisdiction and review them with each client as part of the informed consent process.
- Be cognizant of boundaries in the professional relationship and always consider each client's best interests and treatment needs when crossing professional boundaries.
- Avoid multiple relationships that bring with them the risk of impaired objectivity or conflicts of interest.
- When considering entering into a multiple relationship, consider the client's treatment needs, reasonably available options and alternatives, and the potential risks and benefits of each.
- Make arrangements to ensure that clients are able to access you in between treatment sessions should they experience a crisis.
- During planned absences, make arrangements for emergency coverage with colleagues so that clients' treatment needs will be met.
- Make advance arrangements with a colleague in anticipation of unplanned situations that would prevent you from continuing in practice.
- Do not continue providing treatment when it is not in the client's best interest, such as when the client is not benefitting from treatment or is being harmed by it.
- When terminating professional services, ensure that any ongoing treatment needs are addressed through appropriate referrals.

PRACTICAL RECOMMENDATIONS

- Develop standard routines for discussing availability, emergency procedures, and securing informed consent. Have all clinical staff follow these protocols and communicate them to covering clinicians.
- Develop a policy for dealing with cases involving children and especially divorce and questions of custody, confidentiality, permission to treat the child, and whether or not your work will be available to the court in any pending or future legal action.
- Include directions for dealing with a life-threatening emergency on your voice-mail greeting.
- Discuss multiple relationships that occur, directly and in a timely fashion, and document the outcomes of these discussions in the patient record.
- When building a new practice specialty, be sure to get ongoing clinical supervision and mentoring until your skills are solidified. Then get periodic consultation. Do not assume a weekend or even weeklong course makes you an "expert."
- Err in the direction of caution when providing information to referral sources. What do they need to know? What are you specifically authorized to communicate?

- Seek consultation from trusted mentors if you are unsure about how to best terminate with a client, and then document these discussions in the patient record.

PITFALLS TO AVOID

- Overestimating the boundaries of your clinical competence and inappropriately accepting referrals.
- Allowing fiscal motivations to influence clinical judgment when deciding whether to accept referrals or continue with a client who is not improving.
- Placing potential clients on wait lists without first assessing the appropriateness of doing so, and failing to monitor the status of individuals on a wait list over an extended period of time.
- Assuming clients understand the information shared in the informed consent process without actually assessing their level of understanding.
- Relying on written materials and the client's signature of agreement with these materials rather than carefully reviewing this information with clients verbally.
- Deferring to the parent's or guardian's wishes regarding treatment and excluding minor clients from the information-sharing and decision-making process.
- Failing to negotiate parents' and guardians' rights to treatment information and not giving adequate attention to minor clients' preferences and best interests.
- Failing to fully understand laws in your jurisdiction relevant to mandatory exceptions to confidentiality, and violating the law while endeavoring to acquiesce to client requests for maintaining confidentiality.
- Responding to referral sources' requests for treatment updates and other information without first discussing this with clients and obtaining their informed consent for this sharing of confidential information.
- When authorized to share confidential information with a third party, sharing more than the agreed-upon amount of information and/or more than the minimum amount of information necessary to achieve the goals of the authorized release.
- Failing to anticipate unexpected interruptions to your ability to practice, potentially abandoning clients during a time of significant need.
- Relying on regularly calling in to check voice mail messages during extended periods of absence from practice when clients may be in distress or crisis.
- When utilizing colleagues to provide coverage during periods of planned absence from practice, not carefully screening the appropriateness of these colleagues based on their clinical expertise and availability to serve in this role.

- Taking on an overly rigid policy regarding boundaries and multiple relationships out of a misguided fear of engaging in unethical or harmful behaviors, thus failing to take into consideration client needs and best interests.
- Failing to adequately attend to one's self-care and psychological wellness, allowing professional and personal stressors and demands to contribute to the development of problems of professional competence.
- Engaging in increasingly intrusive boundary crossings and then violations that are motivated by one's own needs and interests, thus overlooking the client's best interests and welfare.
- Continuing to provide treatment when ethically and clinically not warranted out of a fear of charges of client abandonment.
- Failing to provide clients with a termination phase of treatment (pretermination counseling) and not offering to assist them with the referral process when ongoing clinical needs are present.
- Facing ethical dilemmas and challenges independently, relying on one's own judgment and view of the issues, rather than consulting with colleagues and together applying formal models of ethical decision making to determine the most appropriate course of action.
- Not obtaining clinical consultation and input on difficult cases or when faced with an ethical dilemma.

RELEVANT ETHICS CODE STANDARDS

Scope of Practice

- AAMFT Code of Ethics (AAMFT, 2012) Principle 3.2, Knowledge of Regulatory Standards, states, "Marriage and family therapists maintain adequate knowledge of and adhere to applicable laws, ethics, and professional standards" (p. 4), and Principle 3.3, Impairment, states: "Marriage and family therapists seek appropriate professional assistance for their personal problems or conflicts that may impair work performance or clinical judgment" (p. 4).
- ACA Code of Ethics (ACA, 2005) Standard C.2.a, Boundaries of Competence, states, "Counselors gain knowledge, personal awareness, sensitivity, and skills pertinent to working with a diverse client population" (p. 9). It also states in Standard C.2.d., Monitor Effectiveness, "Counselors continually monitor their effectiveness as professionals and take steps to improve when necessary" (p. 9); and in Standard C.2.g., Impairment, it states, "Counselors are alert to the signs of impairment from their own physical, mental, or emotional problems and refrain from offering or providing professional services when such impairment is likely to harm a client or others" (p. 9).

- APA Ethics Code (APA, 2010) Standard 2.01, Boundaries of Competence, states psychologists are guided to "provide services…with populations and in areas only within the boundaries of their competence, based on their education, training, supervised experience, consultation, study or professional experience" (p. 5). APA Ethics Code Standard 2.01d, Boundaries of Competence, states that clinicians may at times need to go beyond the limits of their competence and that "psychologists with closely related prior training or experience may provide such services in order to ensure that services are not denied if they make a reasonable effort to obtain the competence required by using relevant research, training, consultation or study" (p. 5).
- NASW Code of Ethics (NASW, 2008) states in Standard 1.04, Competence, "Social workers should provide services in substantive areas or use intervention techniques or approaches that are new to them only after engaging in appropriate study, training, consultation, and supervision from people who are competent in those interventions or techniques" (p. 2). It also advises in Standard 4.05, Impairment, that when questions of impaired competence arise, social workers "should immediately seek consultation and take appropriate remedial action by seeking professional help, making adjustments in workload, terminating practice, or taking any other steps necessary to protect clients and others" (p. 7).

Clinical Competence and Accepting Referrals

- AAMFT Code of Ethics (AAMFT, 2012) Principle 1.10, Referrals, requires that clinicians "assist persons in obtaining other therapeutic services if the therapist is unable or unwilling, for appropriate reasons, to provide professional help" (p. 3).
- ACA Code of Ethics (ACA, 2005) states, "When counselors transfer or refer clients to other practitioners, they ensure that appropriate clinical and administrative processes are completed and open communication is maintained with both clients and practitioners" (p. 6).
- APA Ethics Code (APA, 2010), Standard 6.07, Referrals and Fees, states, "When psychologists pay, receive payment from or divide fees with another professional, other than in an employer-employee relationship, the payment to each is based on the services provided (clinical, consultative, administrative or other) and is not based on the referral itself" (p. 9).
- NASW Code of Ethics (NASW, 2008) Standard 2.06, Referral for Service, requires that "social workers who refer clients to other professionals should take appropriate steps to facilitate an orderly transfer of responsibility…and should disclose, with clients' consent, all pertinent information to the new service providers" (p. 5).

Informed Consent and Assent

- AAMFT Code of Ethics (AAMFT, 2012) Principle 1.2, Informed Consent, adds that marriage and family therapists must "use language that is reasonably understandable to clients" and that "the content of informed consent may vary depending upon the client and treatment plan" (p. 2).
- ACA Code of Ethics (ACA, 2005) Standard A.2.a, Informed Consent, states that "counselors have an obligation to review in writing and verbally with clients the rights and responsibilities of both the counselor and the client" and that "informed consent is an ongoing part of the counseling process, and counselors appropriately document discussions of informed consent throughout the counseling relationship" (p. 4).
- APA Ethics Code (APA, 2010) Standard 3.10, Informed Consent, requires that prior to any professional service being provided, psychologists "obtain the informed consent of the individual or individuals using language that is reasonably understandable to that person or persons except when conducting such activities without consent is mandated by law or governmental regulation" (p. 6).
- NASW Code of Ethics (NASW, 2008) Standard 1.03, Informed Consent, states that social workers should "protect clients' interests by seeking permission from an appropriate third party, informing clients consistent with the clients' level of understanding. In such instances social workers should seek to ensure that the third party acts in a manner consistent with clients' wishes and interests" (p. 2).

Exceptions to Confidentiality

- AAMFT Code of Ethics (AAMFT, 2012) Principle 2.2, Written Authorization to Release Client Information, states that "Marriage and family therapists do not disclose client confidences except by written authorization or waiver, or where mandated or permitted by law" (p. 3).
- ACA Code of Ethics (ACA, 2005) Standard B.1.d., Explanation of Limits, asserts that counselors are advised to "inform clients of the limitations of confidentiality and seek to identify foreseeable situations in which confidentiality must be breached" (p. 7).
- APA Ethics Code (APA, 2010) Standard 4.02, Discussing Limits of Confidentiality, requires psychologists to review with each client "the relevant limits of confidentiality" and "the foreseeable uses of the information generated through their psychological activities" (p. 7).
- NASW Code of Ethics (NASW, 2008) Standard 1.07, Privacy and Confidentiality, states that "social workers should review with clients circumstances where confidential information may be requested and where disclosure of confidential information may be legally required,"

doing so as early as is feasible and "throughout the course of the
relationship" (p. 3).

Boundaries and Multiple Relationships

- AAMFT Code of Ethics (AAMFT, 2012) Principle 1.3, Multiple
  Relationships, states, "Marriage and family therapists are aware of their
  influential positions with respect to clients, and they avoid exploiting
  the trust and dependency of such persons" and that "when the risk of
  impairment or exploitation exists due to conditions or multiple roles,
  therapists document the appropriate precautions taken" (p. 2).
- ACA Code of Ethics (ACA, 2005) advises in Standard A.5.c.,
  Nonprofessional Interactions or Relationships, that "counselor–client
  nonprofessional relationships with clients, former clients, their romantic
  partners, or their family members should be avoided, except when the
  interaction is potentially beneficial to the client" (p. 5). In such cases,
  counselors are required to engage in these multiple relationships only
  with the client's informed consent after the potential risks and benefits as
  well as options and alternatives are considered, along with the rationale
  for entering into the multiple relationship. Then, if unanticipated negative
  outcomes arise, counselors "must show evidence of an attempt to remedy
  such harm" (p. 5).
- APA Ethics Code (APA, 2010) Standard 3.05, Multiple Relationships,
  makes it clear psychologists are guided to not engage in multiple
  relationships if they "could reasonably be expected to impair the
  psychologist's objectivity, competence or effectiveness in performing
  his or her functions as a psychologist, or otherwise risks exploitation
  or harm to the person with whom the professional relationship exists"
  (p. 6).
- NASW Code of Ethics (NASW, 2008) Standard 1.06b, Conflicts of Interest,
  states, "Social workers should not take unfair advantage of any professional
  relationship or exploit others to further their personal, religious, political,
  or business interests" (p. 3).

Interruptions of Treatment and Addressing Clients' Needs

- AAMFT Code of Ethics (AAMFT, 2012) Principle 1.11,
  Non-Abandonment, states, "Marriage and family therapists do not
  abandon or neglect clients in treatment without making reasonable
  arrangements for the continuation of treatment" (p. 3).
- ACA Code of Ethics (ACA, 2005) requires in Standard A.11.a.,
  Abandonment Prohibited, that "counselors assist in making appropriate

arrangements for the continuation of treatment, when necessary, during interruptions such as vacations, illness, and following termination" (p. 6).

- APA Ethics Code (APA, 2010), Standard 3.12, Interruption of Psychological Services, states that psychologists are advised to "make reasonable efforts to plan for facilitating services in the event that psychological services are interrupted by factors such as the psychologist's illness, death, unavailability, relocation or retirement or by the client's/patient's relocation or financial limitations" (p. 6).
- NASW Code of Ethics (NASW, 2008) Standard 1.15, Interruption of Services, requires that "social workers should make reasonable efforts to ensure continuity of services in the event that services are interrupted by factors such as unavailability, relocation, illness, disability, or death" (p. 4).

Termination and Abandonment

- AAMFT Code of Ethics (AAMFT, 2012) Principle 1.11, Non-Abandonment, states "Marriage and family therapists do not abandon or neglect clients in treatment without making reasonable arrangements for the continuation of such treatment" (p. 3).
- ACA Code of Ethics (ACA, 2005) Standard A.11.a., Abandonment Prohibited, requires that "counselors do not abandon or neglect clients in counseling." (p. 6). It also states in Standard A.11.c., Appropriate Termination, that "counselors terminate a counseling relationship when it becomes reasonably apparent that the client no longer needs assistance, is not likely to benefit, or is being harmed by continued counseling" (p. 6).
- APA Ethics Code (APA, 2010) Standard 10.10, Terminating Therapy, states, "(a) Psychologists terminate therapy when it becomes reasonably clear that the client/patient no longer needs the service, is not likely to benefit, or is being harmed by continued service. (b) Psychologists may terminate therapy when threatened or otherwise endangered by the client/patient or another person with whom the client/patient has a relationship" (p. 13). Additionally, this standard allows that "except where precluded by the actions of clients/patients or third-party payors, prior to termination psychologists provide pretermination counseling and suggest alternative service providers as appropriate" (p. 13).
- NASW Code of Ethics (NASW, 2008) Standard 1.16, Termination of Services, requires that social workers avoid abandoning clients and that they "should withdraw services precipitously only under unusual circumstances, giving careful consideration to all factors in the situation and taking care to minimize possible adverse effects. Social workers should assist in making appropriate arrangements for continuation of services when necessary" (p. 4).

REFERENCES

American Association for Marriage and Family Therapy. (2012). *Code of ethics*. Retrieved from http://www.aamft.org/imis15/content/legal_ethics/code_of_ethics.aspx

American Counseling Association. (2005). *ACA code of ethics*. Retrieved from http://www.counseling.org/Resources/aca-code-of-ethics.pdf

American Psychological Association. (2010). *Ethical principles of psychologists and code of conduct*. Retrieved from http://www.apa.org/ethics

Barnett, J. E., & Walfish, S. (2011). *Billing and collecting for your mental health practice: Effective strategies and ethical practice*. Washington, DC: APA Books.

Barnett, J. E., Doll, B., Younggren, J. N., & Rubin, N. J. (2007). Clinical competence for practicing psychologists: Clearly a work in progress. *Professional Psychology: Research and Practice, 38*(5), 510–517.

Barnett, J. E., & Johnson, W. B. (2009). *Ethics desk reference for counselors*. Alexandria, VA: American Counseling Association.

Barnett, J. E., Wise, E. H., Johnson-Greene, D., & Buckey, S. F. (2007). Informed consent: Too much of a good thing? Or not enough? *Professional Psychology: Research and Practice, 38*(2), 179–186.

Barnett, J. E., & Yutrenzka, B. (1994). Nonsexual dual relationships in professional practice with special applications to rural and military communities. *The Independent Practitioner, 14*(5), 243–248.

Bradley, L. J., Hendricks, B., & Kabell, D. R. (2012). The professional will: An ethical responsibility. *The Family Journal, 2*(3), 309–314.

Brossig, C., & Kalichman, S. (1992). Clinicians' reporting of suspected child abuse: A review of the empirical literature. *Clinical Psychology Review, 12*(2), 155–168.

Brown, C., & Trangsrud, H. B. (2008). Factors associated with acceptance and decline of client gift giving. *Professional Psychology: Research and Practice, 39*(5), 505–511.

Davis, D. A., Mazmanian, P. E., Fordis, M., Harrison, R. V., Thorpe, K. E., & Perrier, L. (2006). Accuracy of physician self-assessment compared with observed measures of competence: A systematic review. *Journal of the American Medical Association, 296*(9), 1094–2009.

Dunning, D., Heath, C., & Suls, J. M. (2004). Flawed self-assessment: Implications for health, education, and the workplace. *Psychological Science in the Public Interest, 5*, 69–106.

Epstein, R. M., & Hundert, E. M. (2002). Defining and assessing professional competence. *Journal of the American Medical Association, 287*(2), 226–235.

Erickson Cornish, J. A., Schreier, B. A., Nadkarni, L. I., Metzger, L. H., & Rodolfa, E. R. (Eds.). (2010). *Handbook of multicultural counseling competencies*. Hoboken, NJ: Wiley.

Eva, K. W., Cunnington, J. P. W., Reiter, H. I., Keane, D. R., & Norman, G. R. (2004). How can I know what I don't know? Poor self assessment in a well-defined domain. *Advances in Health Sciences Education, 9*, 211–224.

Firestone, R., & Barnett, J. E. (2012). The ethical practice of psychology in rural settings. *The Independent Practitioner, 32*(3), 102–106.

Fisher, C. B., & Oransky, M. (2008). Informed consent to psychotherapy: Protecting dignity and respecting the autonomy of patients. *Journal of Clinical Psychology, 64*(5), 576–588.

Gottlieb, M. C., & Younggren, J. N. (2009). Is there a slippery slope? Considerations regarding multiple relationships and risk management. *Professional Psychology: Research and Practice, 40*(6), 564–571.

Gutheil, T. G., & Gabbard, G. O. (1993). The concept of boundaries in clinical practice: Theoretical and risk-management dimensions. *The American Journal of Psychiatry, 150*(2), 188–196.

Jobes, D. A, Overholser, J. C., Rudd, M. D., & Joiner, T. E. (2008). Ethical and competent care of suicidal patients: Contemporary challenges, new developments, and considerations for clinical practice. *Professional Psychology: Research and Practice, 39*(4), 405–413.

Kalichman, S., & Craig, M. (1991). Professional psychologists' decisions to report suspected child abuse: Clinician and situation influences. *Professional Psychology: Research and Practice, 22*(1), 84–89.

Koocher, G. P. (2007). All in the family. In J. E. Barnett, S. Behnke, S. L. Rosenthal, & G. P. Koocher, In case of ethical dilemma break glass: Commentary on ethical decision making in practice. *Professional Psychology: Research and Practice, 38*(1), 7–12.

Kuther, T. L. (2003). Medical decision-making and minors: Issues of consent and assent. *Adolescence, 39*(150), 343–358.

National Association of Social Workers. (2008). *Code of ethics.* Retrieved from http://www.socialworkers.org/pubs/code/code.asp

Schank, J., Helbok, C. M., Haldeman, D. C., & Gallardo, M. E. (2010). Challenges and benefits of ethical small-community practice. *Professional Psychology: Research and Practice, 41*(6), 502–510.

Shapiro, D. L., & Smith, S. R. (2011). Confidentiality and privacy. In D. L. Shapiro & S. R. Smith (Eds.), *Malpractice in psychology: A practical resource for clinicians* (pp. 61–77). Washington, DC: American Psychological Association.

Smith, D., & Fitzpatrick, M. (1995). Patient-therapist boundary issues: An integrative review of theory and research. *Professional Psychology: Research and Practice, 26*(5), 499–506.

State of Maryland. Health General Article § 20-104. *Mental or emotional disorder.* Retrieved from http://dhmh.maryland.gov/psych/SitePages/lawsregs.aspx

Tarasoff v. Regents of the University of California, 551 P.2d 334 (Cal 1976) vacating and modifying 529 P.2d 553 (Cal 1974).

Vasquez, M. J. T. (2007). Sometimes a taco is just a taco. In J. E. Barnett, A. A. Lazarus, M. J. T. Vasquez, O. Moorehead-Slaughter, & W. B. Johnson, Boundary issues and multiple relationships: Fantasy and reality. *Professional Psychology: Research and Practice, 38*(4), 401–410.

Vasquez, M. J. T., Bingham, R. P., & Barnett, J. E. (2008). Psychotherapy termination: Clinical and ethical responsibilities. *Journal of Clinical Psychology: In Session, 64*(5), 653–665.

Walfish, S., & Barnett, J. (2009) *Financial success in mental health practice: Essential tools and strategies for practitioners.* Washington DC: APA Books.

Walfish, S., McAllister, B., O'Connell, P., & Lambert, M. (2012) An investigation of self-assessment bias in mental health providers. *Psychological Reports, 110*(2), 639–644.

Werth, J., Welfel, E., & Benjamin, G. A. (2008) *The duty to protect: Ethical, legal, and professional considerations for mental health professionals.* Washington, DC: APA Books.

Younggren, J. N., Fisher, M. A., Foote, W. E., & Hjelt, S. E. (2011). A legal and ethi-
cal review of patient responsibilities and psychotherapist duties. *Professional Psychology: Research and Practice*, *42*(2), 160–68.

Younggren, J. N., & Gottlieb, M. C. (2004). Managing risk when contemplating multiple relationships. *Professional Psychology: Research and Practice*, *35*(3), 255–260.

Zur, O. (2007). *Boundaries in psychotherapy*. Washington, DC: American Psychological Association.

SAMPLE TERMINATION LETTER

Steven Walfish, Ph.D.
2004 Cliff Valley Way, Suite 101
Atlanta, Georgia 30329
(404) 728-0728

August 30, 2013
Jane Doe
127 Main Street
Anywhere, USA

Re: Stopping Counseling

Dear Ms. Doe:

I hope things are going well for you. Please know that you missed our last appointment that was scheduled for August 15th at 4 p.m. I attempted to reach you by telephone, but you did not respond to the voice message I left. Since I have not heard back from you to schedule another counseling appointment I am assuming that you want to stop counseling at this time.

If I do not hear back from you within two weeks I will consider our work together in counseling to be completed. Please be aware that if you would like to resume sessions with me that you are welcome to contact me in the future. However, I cannot guarantee that I will have openings in my schedule at that time. If you would like to resume counseling, but for any reason would prefer to work with another counselor, please consider contacting your Primary Care Physician for a referral, or use the Find a Psychologist Directory on the website of the Georgia Psychological Association (www.gapsychology.com).

It is important to ensure that your use of any prescribed medication is closely monitored by your prescribing physician. Further, you should take your medication as it is prescribed and follow up immediately with your prescribing physician if any increased difficulties or side effects are experienced. If you experience any crises or emergency situations you should contact your prescribing physician or your Primary Care Physician, or call 9-1-1 or go to the nearest emergency room immediately.

I wish you success in your future endeavors. Please feel free to let me know if I may be of any further assistance to you.

Sincerely,
Steven Walfish, Ph.D.
Licensed Psychologist

3

Documentation and
Record Keeping

Most mental health professionals do not get excited when they hear the words "documentation and record keeping." In fact, many may groan and think of this as an onerous burden—a necessary evil that comes along with the more enjoyable and rewarding activity of working with clients. Yet documentation and record keeping are essential and important elements of competent, ethical, and effective clinical treatment. Additionally, as will be seen, the timely, relevant, and thoughtful documentation of the clinical services we provide is good business practice.

DOCUMENTATION

Many mental health professionals may question why we need to document the clinical services we provide, and perhaps even struggle with just how to document: how much detail to include, how extensive to make each note, what wording to use, and what issues to include or exclude from the notes made. It is our belief that being aware of the many purposes of documentation and record keeping will be invaluable in guiding the mental health professional in how to carry out documentation and record keeping duties.

Although each of these will not necessarily apply in every situation, possible purposes of documentation and record keeping (Barnett, 2000) include the following.

Assisting You in Providing Ongoing Treatment in a Competent and Effective Manner

No professional will be able to remember all the details of every client's treatment, their history, their presenting problems, issues discussed in past sessions, homework assignments given, and the like. Being able to refer back to previous treatment-session notes can prove invaluable for refreshing your memory and not forgetting or overlooking relevant treatment information. Those with busy practices and many clients will find this to be especially important.

Assisting You If a Client Returns to Treatment at a Later Date

Many clients leave treatment for a period of time and then return. Clients typically leave treatment when their goals have been achieved. However, if they have found the services you provided to be valuable when experiencing new challenges, difficulties, or important life transitions, they will view you as an important resource and seek help. Having access to past treatment notes, when they contain relevant treatment information, can prove very helpful to client and psychotherapist alike. This can help ensure the most efficient and effective use of the client's and psychotherapist's time during treatment sessions. Clients also appreciate "being remembered" and not feeling like they have to start all over by retelling their story.

Assisting Other Professionals When a Client's Treatment Is Transferred

At times, it may be in a client's best interest to be transferred to the care of a different clinician. This may occur when the client's treatment needs change or when these needs exceed the mental health professional's areas of competence. Providing the new clinician with information about past treatment can prove invaluable for having an understanding of the client's difficulties and creating the new treatment plan. This may also occur if you become unavailable or incapacitated, or die. We must consider these possibilities and realize that our documentation may be the only way to communicate with the new treating professional.

Assisting Future Treating Professionals

Clients who move their place of residence may enter treatment with someone new. Some clients who decide to enter treatment again at a future date may choose to work with a different mental health professional. Being able to forward past treatment records can be of great benefit to the new clinician in developing the client's treatment plan. Understanding the course of past treatment, challenges experienced, techniques and strategies used, and outcomes achieved can all be useful information for the new clinician, and therefore of benefit to the client.

An Important Form of Communication Among Members of a Treatment Team

Many mental health treatment facilities function with a team treatment approach, such as those practicing in an interdisciplinary setting. Often an integrated or holistic treatment approach is most effective for clients. This may become even more commonplace with the advent of standardized electronic medical records. Each team member's documentation of services provided, and contacts with clients, can be of great assistance to other team members who are working with the client. Knowing, for example, that a client experienced a relationship loss, was in an altercation with another client, or attempted suicide over the weekend would be valuable information for other team members to know before their next meeting with the client.

As a Risk Management Strategy

It is widely accepted that the documentation of the professional services we provide is the tangible record of our good-faith efforts to meet our profession's standard of care. Should an ethics committee or licensing board complaint ever be filed, or charges of malpractice ever arise, it will be our documentation that is examined for evidence of the professional services provided, decisions made, factors considered, the client's level of participation and cooperation, any consultations that occurred, and more. In essence, our documentation will be used to determine the quality of professional services provided, but it must be made contemporaneously with the services provided to be considered valid.

For Insurance Purposes

When clients are utilizing their health insurance to provide coverage for the mental health services they obtain, insurance companies and MCOs will often require some level of documentation as part of their utilization review process. Failure to maintain adequate documentation that includes assessments and diagnoses, describes the treatment plan, shows that the sessions reflect working on these stated treatment goals, and delineates the services provided and demonstrates outcomes achieved can result in services not being reimbursed. If services were reimbursed, a retrospective review may result in the insurer asking for (and likely being entitled to, based on the agreed upon contract) a refund of monies already paid for services.

Because It Is the Law and Your Profession's Code of Ethics Requires It

The code of ethics of every mental health profession, and the laws and regulations that pertain to the practice of these professions, require that we document all professional services we provide. At a minimum this tends to include assessments and test results, diagnoses, treatment provided, consultations, client contacts as well as those with others about the client and information obtained, recommendations made, the outcomes of interventions and the client's level of cooperation (e.g., client does not follow through with treatment recommendations or complete homework assignments, frequently cancels or misses appointments, does not take medication as prescribed, etc.), the disposition of the client and referrals made, and how and when termination occurred.

HOW TO DOCUMENT

So, how should we document? How much information is sufficient, how much is too much, and how should it be worded? Key points to keep in mind include the following.

Write With the Potential Uses of These Records in Mind

When documenting, keep in mind that these are not you own personal or private notes. Others may be reading them at a later date (whether it be future treating professionals who base their treatment plan on your past treatment, to demonstrate the quality of the services you provided in response to a malpractice suit that has been filed against you, etc.). Include information relevant to the possible future uses of these records.

Write With the Intended Audience in Mind

Do not use jargon, shorthand abbreviations, or phrases that only you understand. Further, if notes are handwritten, ensure that they are legible. Write using objective statements and observations rather than including subjective opinions or judgments. You want the reader to be able to picture what transpired in treatment, what each party's role was, and what outcomes were achieved. For example, consider what a colleague filling in for you during a period of unanticipated absence would need to know about past treatment sessions. Similarly, what would you want a licensing board that is investigating a complaint against you to read? Keep in mind that the adage "if it isn't written, it didn't happen" is typically the standard used by those evaluating our documentation. Further, they may also have the perspective that "the quality of the documentation is representative of the quality of the professional services provided."

Create Treatment Records in a Timely Manner

We all know the effects of the passage of time on memory. But, if you are not sure, try waiting a day or a week and then document a day's worth of psychotherapy sessions. See how the passage of time affects the quality of the notes you write to include the amount of detail. We recommend that all documentation occur immediately after the conclusion of the treatment session, if at all possible. If documentation must be done at a later date, we recommend that, in addition to recording the date and time of the session, that the date and time when the documentation occurred be included as well.

Only Include Information Relevant to the Client's Treatment

Remembering that others are likely to read the treatment records we create, we recommend that only information relevant to the treatment being provided be included in the notes. Clients may share incidental information or make offhand comments that are not relevant to their treatment goals or the treatment provided, and that might be embarrassing or even harmful if others were to have access to this information. Additionally, it is important to release the information that you have personally produced, not information that was sent to you or obtained from other sources.

Include All Relevant Materials in the Client's Record

In addition to treatment session notes, this may include the informed consent agreement, HIPAA Notice of Privacy Practices, a financial agreement, insurance paperwork and treatment plans, any assessments conducted to include test protocols and results, communications with the client and with others about the client, telephone messages, copies of e-mail communications, and any materials the client may have given to you, such as personal writings.

Be Guided by Your Profession's Code of Ethics, Your Licensing Law and Relevant Regulations, and Applicable Professional Guidelines

Each of these documents will provide guidance and minimal standards for clinical documentation. For example, all psychologists should consider the guidance provided in the APA's Record Keeping Guidelines (APA, 2007). Although these are not enforceable minimal standards that must always be met (like licensing laws, regulations, and codes of ethics), they provide useful guidance on how to document and what to include in our documentation.

In keeping these points in mind, you will encounter times when clients ask you not to keep a record or not to put something in a record. This often happens with "high profile" clients and with other clients who are concerned about the possible breach of the record's confidentiality. At other times, it occurs when clients are seeing the clinician for consultation and do not view themselves as having established a doctor–patient relationship (e.g., parents seeking one session for input about their child, an executive getting coaching from the clinician, a patient who writes a letter to the clinician). It is our recommendation that it is an ethical (and risk management) imperative that a record is opened on all clients who receive services and that all pertinent information be included in that record (including records of phone calls and thank-you notes from clients). Documentation needs to represent the complete set of interactions with the client, whether they are receiving health care or other professional services.

FINANCIAL RECORDS

In addition to creating, securely storing, and maintaining clinical records for each client, mental health professionals should do the same with financial records as well. Financial records should be created separately for each client and should include their identifying information, the date of each service provided, the service provided, who provided the service, the amount of time spent providing the service, the fee charged for the service, if payment was received, and the form and amount of payment. These financial records should be maintained for the same amount of time that clinical records are maintained in accordance with relevant law.

USE OF TECHNOLOGY AND ELECTRONIC HEALTH RECORDS

The use of technology in documentation and record keeping, and electronic health records (EHR) in particular, provide mental health professionals with both opportunities and challenges (Richards, 2009). Opportunities include the ease of creating, storing, and accessing records. Additionally, members of treatment teams and health care networks have greatly increased access to assessment and treatment records, to create and update records as well as to access them when providing treatment.

Challenges associated with the use of technology and EHR include controlling access to the records and protecting their security, maintaining the integrity of the records, and ensuring that they are adequately backed up. Relevant concerns include unauthorized access to EHR and the inadvertent release of confidential information, whether by human error or by security violations.

It is vital that mental health professionals who use technology to create, store, and disseminate records do so with the protection of each client's confidentiality in mind, and that they develop security policies and procedures and ensure that these are adhered to by all subordinates. These may include never taking a laptop containing client information out of the office, ensuring that all computers are password protected with passwords being complex combinations of letters, numbers, and other characters to minimize the risk of hackers accessing the records, and ensuring that all computer systems have virus and malware protection that is kept up to date (Barnett & Scheetz, 2003). See Chapter 4 for a more detailed description of some of these security practices.

RECORDS WHEN MORE THAN ONE PERSON IS BEING TREATED

Many mental health professionals provide treatment to couples, families, and groups. Each of these creates documentation and record-keeping challenges. In group treatment the widely accepted practice is to create a separate treatment record for each group member. Doing so helps to protect the privacy of each member. Further, when it is appropriate to mention another group member in a client's record, it is recommended that the other client's initials be used, again to protect privacy.

When treating couples and families, it may be viewed that the couple or family is "the client." Accordingly, one treatment record is typically created. But because one person may not waive privilege for another, it is important to address in the informed consent process that permission will be needed from all parties before the record may be released.

RECORD KEEPING, STORAGE, AND DISPOSAL

Once the clinical record has been created, it must be stored and maintained in accordance with the relevant code of ethics standards and with relevant laws and regulations in your jurisdiction. Key issues to consider when deciding how to store records include accessibility of the records by you and by others authorized to have access to them, and security of the records to prevent unauthorized access to them. Additionally, records must be maintained for at least the minimum amount of time specified in your jurisdiction's relevant law or regulation, as well as the length of time cited by the applicable guidelines (whichever is longer), and when records are disposed of, they must be destroyed in a manner that ensures that each client's confidentiality is maintained, such as by shredding. Just crumbling or ripping up records is not sufficient and can lead to ethics and HIPAA violations.

WHAT HAPPENS WHEN A CLIENT IS DECEASED

It is understood that each individual client has the legal right to decide if his or her record should be released. When a client dies, however, this creates what may be seen as a dilemma. It is unlikely that most mental health professionals will include provisions for such an occurrence in their informed consent process. Mental health professionals nevertheless should be familiar with relevant laws in their jurisdiction that address this issue. Typically, the executor of the client's estate becomes the holder of privilege of the deceased client's records. Consulting with an attorney in these situations is recommended, especially because the executor may have intentions for release or distribution of the records that are inconsistent with your understanding of the client's wishes. Again, this is a legal issue, so consulting an attorney in these situations is recommended. Before releasing records it is also essential to inspect the paperwork and make sure that it is indeed valid. It is also advisable to inform the executor of the pros and cons of releasing the information. Informed consent plays a role here as well. One of the authors had the experience of a sibling claiming they were the responsible administrator of the estate and getting an order compelling release, when the spouse was actually the executor. A call to the spouse (before the information was released) discussing the order that was received led to the matter being cleared up by the attorneys and the deceased patient's confidentiality being protected.

Ethically, mental health professionals are guided to consider their former client's wishes. Commentators in the professional literature (e.g., Werth, Burke, & Bardash, 2002) propose that confidentiality survives the client and records should be released only in the most unusual circumstances, such as when public safety may be at risk. No clear case law or ethics guidance exists at present on this issue, and mental health professionals are guided to give careful consideration to the ethics and legal issues involved when making decisions about releasing a deceased client's records.

As is emphasized throughout the mental health professions' codes of ethics, the application of the requirements of these codes must be considered in the context of relevant laws and regulations in your jurisdiction. We recommend that mental health professionals remain cognizant of what is required by relevant laws and what is allowed under the law. When conflicts between laws or regulations and the code of ethics arise, we recommend that the standard most protective of clients' rights and welfare be selected.

ETHICAL CHALLENGES

- Providing the right amount of detail in your documentation. There is no formula for how much and what type of information to include. We must exercise our judgment, keeping in mind who may have access to the records as well as the possible uses of the records.
- Remembering information at a later time or date and wanting to add it to the treatment record. Never try to add additional information to a treatment record at a later time or date in a manner that makes it appear that you wrote this when doing the original documentation. Make an addendum to the note, indicating the date and time the new information was added.

- Providing administrative staff and subordinates with adequate training and oversight. It is important to remember that most administrative staff will not have training in ethics relevant to the mental health professions. Teach staff the importance of seeking consultation with you should they have even the slightest doubt or question about confidentiality.
- Deciding on the level of security precautions needed to sufficiently safeguard records. Do not underestimate security needs and do not have a lax attitude or approach to addressing them.
- Making advance arrangements in anticipation of unavailability, incapacitation, or death. It is important that needed arrangements be made, such as a professional will, so that clients will have access to their records even if one of these circumstances arises.

KEY POINTS TO KEEP IN MIND

- Record keeping should not be viewed as a "chore" or something that increases your exposure if a claim or complaint is filed against you. It serves many useful purposes, including offering you a better defense against a complaint, compared to having sparse or no records.
- It is essential to know your jurisdiction's requirements and your profession-specific standards regarding record keeping. These may change over time as standards and statutes change and as technology plays more of a role in your practice.
- You are responsible for the security of your records regardless of whether you own the practice or work for someone else. You also are responsible for the behaviors of the administrative staff when it comes to the security of the record (even if administratively they do not report to you).
- Rarely is a request for information an actual emergency. You should respond in a timely fashion, but you do not have to rush. Consider your actions carefully. Do you have truly informed consent from the client or responsible party? Are you releasing the information required? Are you inappropriately releasing some information (e.g., information that was sent to you by other sources)?
- Do not simply trust what an attorney requesting or demanding information asserts.
- Develop a relationship with an attorney who is familiar with the relevant statutes in your jurisdiction, and when in doubt consult with that attorney about the legal requirements of the request. Similarly, consult with a trusted mentor about the ethical implications related to the request and how to best address the client's interests as you consider your options.

PRACTICAL RECOMMENDATIONS

- Store all records securely, such as in a fire-retardant file cabinet that is kept locked at all times. Keep the key to the file cabinet in a secure location and do not leave it out in plain sight or in a place where it can easily be found (e.g., under your desk phone).
- If possible, access to the room that records are stored in should be restricted as well.
- Establish written record-keeping policies and procedures. Ensure that all staff members, subordinates, and colleagues in your practice are informed about them, trained to follow them, and that they act in accordance with them. Take personal responsibility for ensuring that this happens. Even solo practitioners are required by HIPAA to have these policies.
- Provide adequate oversight of administrative staff. After training them on record-keeping policies and procedures, have them sign an agreement or contract that stipulates specific ethics requirements they must follow, such as the steps necessary to protect and preserve each client's confidentiality. Ensure that staff members understand that this is a requirement of their job.
- Never leave records lying around unsecured and unattended. This includes leaving the client's name exposed when files are sitting on your desk.
- Take special care if considering bringing a record out of the office to work on for any reason.
- When using EHR or storing confidential information on a computer, be sure to use appropriate safeguards, including virus and malware protection as well as encryption.
- Always back up all materials stored electronically to ensure that records are not lost if a technological problem occurs. It is advisable to have two backups, one onsite and one offsite.
- Safeguard all electronically stored materials by the use of a password that is changed every several months and that is sufficiently long and complex to thwart the efforts of hackers.
- Do not dispose of records prior to the minimum time since the date of last professional contact with the client that is allowed by law.
- Record retention laws provide the minimum amount of time for maintaining records before they may be destroyed. But there often are times when records should be maintained beyond this date, such as with assessment results that provide baseline information on the client's functioning and when further treatment in the future is likely.
- When disposing of records, do so in a manner that preserves the confidentiality of the records such as by shredding. When using commercial shredding vendors, be present to observe the shredding process to ensure the records are destroyed and that confidentiality is maintained.

- When disposing of electronic devices that store clinical information, be sure to destroy the storage drive(s). Simply deleting the information may not sufficiently erase it from the system.
- Be careful about keeping last names and e-mail addresses of clients on your electronic devices, as these may be inadvertently uploaded to the Internet if you subscribe to some social media sites.

PITFALLS TO AVOID

- Failing to document all services provided.
- Failing to document in a timely manner.
- Creating illegible notes.
- Using subjective statements, jargon, and shorthand.
- Not including sufficient information or detail.
- Providing too much detail and irrelevant information.
- Not keeping the potential uses of the documentation in mind when creating it.
- Taking short cuts by using simple or easily guessed passwords.
- Leaving confidential records accessible to unauthorized parties even "for just a few minutes."
- Not updating your virus and malware protection periodically.
- Bringing confidential records home and leaving them unattended and unsecured.
- Leaving confidential material in your car while running an errand.
- Not providing sufficient training and oversight to administrative staff.
- Leaving files laying on your desk so that clients can read the identity of other clients.
- Failing to make a professional will and not keeping it up to date.
- Not being familiar with and following relevant laws and regulations.

RELEVANT ETHICS CODE STANDARDS

Documentation of Professional Services

- AAMFT Code of Ethics (AAMFT, 2012) Principle 3.6, Maintenance of Records, states, "Marriage and family therapists maintain accurate and adequate clinical and financial records in accordance with applicable law" (p. 4).
- ACA Code of Ethics (ACA, 2005) Standard B.6.e., Assistance with Records, states, "When clients request access to their records, counselors provide assistance and consultation in interpreting counseling records" (p. 8); and in Standard B.6.d., Client Access, "Counselors limit the access of clients to

their records, or portions of their records, only when there is compelling
evidence that such access would cause harm to the client" (p. 8).

- APA Ethics Code (APA, 2010) Standard 6.01, Documentation of
Professional and Scientific Work and Maintenance of Records, requires
psychologists to document all professional services "in order to
(1) facilitate provision of services later by them or by other professionals,
(2) allow for replication of research design and analyses, (3) meet
institutional requirements, (4) ensure accuracy of billing and payments,
and (5) ensure compliance with law" (p. 9).

- NASW Code of Ethics (NASW, 2008) Standard 1.08, Access to Records,
states, "Social workers should provide clients with reasonable access
to records concerning the clients" and "When providing clients with
access to their records, social workers should take steps to protect the
confidentiality of other individuals identified or discussed in such records"
(p. 4).

Record Retention, Storage, and Disposal

- AAMFT Code of Ethics (AAMFT, 2012) Principle 2.4, Protection of
Records, requires that "Marriage and family therapists store, safeguard,
and dispose of client records in ways that maintain confidentiality and in
accord with applicable laws and professional standards" (p. 3).

- ACA Code of Ethics (ACA, 2005) Standard B.6.g., Storage and Disposal
After Termination, requires that "counselors store records following
termination of services to ensure reasonable future access, maintain
records in accordance with local and federal statutes governing records,
and dispose of client records and other sensitive materials in a manner that
protects client confidentiality" (p. 8).

- APA Ethics Code (APA, 2010) Standard 6.01, Documentation of
Professional and Scientific Work and Maintenance of Records, requires
psychologists to exercise caution as they "maintain, disseminate, store,
retain and dispose of records and data relating to their professional
and scientific work" (p. 9). Further, Standard 6.02, Maintenance,
Dissemination, and Disposal of Confidential Records of Professional
and Scientific Work, requires psychologists to "maintain confidentiality
in creating, storing, accessing, transferring and disposing of records
under their control, whether these are written, automated or in any other
medium" (p. 9).

- NASW Code of Ethics (NASW, 2008) Standard 3.04, Client Records, states,
"Social workers should store records following the termination of services
to ensure reasonable future access. Records should be maintained for the
number of years required by jurisdiction's statutes or relevant contracts"
(p. 6).

REFERENCES

American Association for Marriage and Family Therapy. (2012). *Code of ethics*. Retrieved from http://www.aamft.org/imis15/content/legal_ethics/code_of_ethics.aspx

American Counseling Association. (2005). *ACA code of ethics*. Retrieved from http://www.counseling.org/Resources/aca-code-of-ethics.pdf

American Psychological Association. (2007). Record keeping guidelines. *American Psychologist*, *62*(9), 993–1004. Retrieved from http://www.apa.org/practice/guidelines/record-keeping.pdf

American Psychological Association. (2010). *Ethical principles of psychologists and code of conduct*. Retrieved from http://www.apa.org/ethics

Barnett, J. E. (December, 2000). Document This! *42 Online. The online journal of Psychologists in Independent Practice, a division of the American Psychological Association*. Retrieved from http://www.division42.org/

Barnett, J. E., & Scheetz, K. (2003). Technological advances and telehealth: Ethics, law, and the practice of psychology. *Psychotherapy: Theory/Research/Practice/Training*, *40*, 86–93.

National Association of Social Workers. (2008). *Code of ethics*. Retrieved from http://www.socialworkers.org/pubs/code/code.asp

Richards, M. M. (2009). Electronic medical records: Confidentiality issues in the time of HIPAA. *Professional Psychology: Research and Practice*, *40*(6), 550–556. doi:10.1037/a0016853

Werth, J. L., Burke, C., & Bardash, R. J. (2002). Confidentiality in end-of-life and after-death situations. *Ethics & Behavior*, *12*(3), 205–222.

4

Dealing With Third Parties and Protecting Confidentiality

In our experience, most mental health professionals are by nature and training concerned about confidentiality. Usually they do not knowingly and intentionally share confidential client information with other individuals. Yet breaches of confidentiality seem to occur relatively frequently and can easily result in potential harm to a client and a complaint against one's license. We believe that many such breaches are caused by a combination of factors, including but not limited to poor attention to detail, the absence of or failure to follow routine policies and procedures, a loss of focus on one's own behavior as it relates to maintaining confidentiality, and behaving with good intentions but in a way that falls outside of accepted standards of care. In this chapter we first focus on general policies when dealing with third parties to avoid ethical mishaps. We then discuss some special situations and options for how they may best be handled. Concepts and approaches related to confidentiality, as well as other interactions with third parties, also will be addressed.

GENERAL POLICIES

Establish Clear Information Protocols for Self and Staff Members

Building sound habits and protocols goes a long way to avoiding unintended breaches. Even the solo practitioner can and should have procedures for routine tasks, such as releasing information from a client's file. Having such protocols in place can be especially helpful when you are overwhelmed, anxious, or stressed. They can help you avoid responding carelessly or out of emotional tension or frustration. Developing routines for sharing information and checking to make sure that all necessary steps have been taken to avoid unintended breaches can go a long way to getting it right more often than not.

Write down your policies for securing protected health information. These should not be things that are just passed on from one person to the next. You cannot always trust that they will remember every detail, either in their initial instruction or years later. Take the administration of your practice seriously and build reference sheets and policies. Even if you are in solo practice, these can be helpful tools, especially when you are rushed or pressured or when there is a formal or informal complaint, because you can point to and follow your written policies.

Be Clear About HIPAA and Your Local Regulatory Requirements

HIPAA requirements regarding confidentiality represent the minimum requirements imposed on health care providers. State law and regulations may have other requirements that exceed the HIPAA standards and need to be respected. For example, HIPAA may authorize that two healthcare providers can exchange information on a common patient without a release if they believe it is in the best interest of the client. However, state law may include a more restrictive standard and require a signed release from the client before sharing information. Similarly, HIPAA may exclude the release of what they term "Process Notes." However, if you are deposed you may indeed be required to release any and all information in your possession about a client. Be sure to carefully read your state laws and regulations regarding confidentiality. Sometimes this is embedded in the licensing law. Read the definitions associated with the statute, as they can specify who it covers. We also recommend completing a HIPAA-specific training workshop to synthesize the relevant information that you need to attend to, be familiar with, and apply in the day-to-day conduct of your practice.

Explain the Limits to Confidentiality at the Outset of Treatment

It is likely that patients will assume that what they say is completely confidential. Yet this is not the case. A mandatory aspect of informed consent is explaining the limits of confidentiality. At the outset of the very first session it is essential to discuss a few "administrative details" and specifically address the situations in which confidentiality is not maintained (e.g., danger to self or others, child or elder abuse, when you have a judge's order to testify, when treatment or an evaluation are court-ordered or required by a third party, or when the client or responsible party has signed a release). Providing this education before the client begins to discuss their personal information can help avoid a situation in which the client did not have a clear understanding of what you might not be able to hold confidential (e.g., the client admitting that they recently pushed and hurt a child or elderly parent). You should routinely train your clinical staff to understand the limits of confidentiality as well. It can be helpful to place your informed consent agreements on your website so that you can encourage clients to read them prior to the first session. If you do not have a website, you can mail or e-mail these documents to the client (with permission) before the first meeting.

Obtaining Informed Consent to Release Information

One key issue when it comes to confidentiality is that of informed consent. It is our obligation to actively ensure that our clients understand what they are agreeing to when they enter treatment or an evaluation process and any implications and risks relevant to this agreement. It is not sufficient merely to have a signature on a form. That may be consent, but it is not *informed* consent.

Many health care settings and lawyers may have your patient sign a blank release form that later gets filled in and sent to you with your name on it. This way the entity requesting information from you can have the individual sign one form and repeatedly reuse that form when seeking information from a variety of sources. A signed release form does not necessarily mean that the patient has specifically given you permission to release the information. At times, you may receive a release that specifically allows another professional to contact you (e.g., another psychotherapist), but does not explicitly allow you to speak to that professional. Be extremely vigilant to make sure you have appropriate documentation and follow only what the client has given you permission to do. For example, if the client wants you both to provide information to and receive it from another party, the release should be worded as such. If they only want you to provide information to the third party, this too must be stated on the release.

The patient may not know what specific information is being requested or how it might be used. You should be sure that the patient (or responsible party) and others present are fully informed about the risks and benefits of sharing information (i.e., *informed* consent). For example, you have been treating a patient for depression and anxiety for some time. The patient decides to sue their employer for wrongful termination. The patient's lawyer asks for records that also include a description of the patient's traumatic childhood history. The patient may be under the impression that their lawyer simply "needs" the records and may not understand that through the legal process of discovery, these records, including the traumatic history (and all the details documented in the treatment record), may be released to the employer's attorney and then be used against the patient in a subsequent trial. Transcripts of court proceedings usually become public record. It is your obligation to make sure the patient understands what is going to be disclosed, how it might be used, and the potential implications for the patient of these uses of their private information.

Additionally, you need to make sure that you have sought out all the appropriate parties who need to waive privilege. One adult party cannot waive privilege for another. For example, John Smith's attorney requests the complete file. John was the patient of record two years ago. However, marital treatment was provided. What the lawyer did not mention in the cover letter to the request for records is that John and Mary are now in a contentious divorce battle and the records are being sought to support John's claims for custody. In instances of couple or family therapy, information may be wrongly disclosed even though the patient of record signed the release. It is important to make sure that other family members have also given their informed consent to release the information (including partners or other guardians when legally required to do so).

It is crucial to read a release carefully to make sure it appropriately authorizes you to provide information and to determine what information is being requested. For example a release may request all psychological information related to the patient. If you are not a psychologist, one might argue that you do not have that information. Similarly, if the release is related to the patient and you have provided marital work, or you saw both an adolescent patient and their parent, the release may not be valid without the signed release by all who were present. In fact, a release signed by a parent for an adolescent who is no longer a minor may not be a legally valid request. The former adolescent who has now reached the age of majority should be contacted to sign their own authorization to allow you to release the information. They have the legal right to decide whether or not to release their mental health records.

You should also directly check with the client to make sure they have indeed authorized the release of information and that they understand the purpose of the release, its risks and benefits, and how in a worst case scenario the release may impact the client (including your professional relationship with the client). There have been many instances where the authors have actually had clients rescind a release after such a frank discussion. You might be interested in developing a checklist to help make sure the release is indeed appropriate, informed, and valid (see sample at the end of this chapter).

Deal Carefully With Legal Requests and Demands

Many attorneys take a reasonable, transparent, and collegial approach with mental health professionals. However, there are others who are not transparent and still others who are demanding and can be threatening and possibly abusive. We have had an experience in which an attorney provided false information about the nature of a subpoena (as opposed to a court order) and did not inform opposing counsel they were demanding records. Upon learning of this, the opposing counsel filed a complaint with the State Bar against the attorney for being misleading with a psychologist and not providing appropriate notice. Be sure you completely understand whom the attorney represents, to what the request pertains, and how the release of your records or your testimony may put the client at risk. You cannot allow yourself to act out of fear or intimidation by attorneys who may use heavy-handed techniques. We have also had the experience of a demand to attend a deposition and produce a client's personal information. Upon obtaining legal counsel, we were immediately informed that the deposition was not in order and did not meet the requirements of notice. Additionally, the clinician could not be compelled legally to produce the information being requested. In essence, the subpoena seemed to be a heavy-handed scare tactic that only another attorney could ascertain. Responding without legal input could have led to the psychologist to attend the deposition and, out of ignorance, release information that rightfully should not be produced. It is important to note that some malpractice policies will cover hiring an attorney to help you combat a subpoena for a deposition to which you object.

It is also important to understand that in many instances you are not free to pick and choose what information is withheld from the attorney. Often in the legal arena the concept of a limited release (where you only provide some of the file) does not apply. This can leave the client open to being in a compromised situation when information that is in their treatment record can be used by an opposing attorney in a way that is detrimental to the client's position in the case. You must assume that whatever information you provide to the client's attorney will also be accessible to the attorney for the opposing side. If you're not sure about releasing the information, take your time and seek input from colleagues, your malpractice carrier, and possibly your own attorney. Then carefully assess your options. Don't hesitate to discuss the risks of releasing the information with your client (and possibly in front of the judge if you are ordered into court).

If you have concerns about the advisability of releasing the information, consider saying the following to a patient's attorney who is making a demand: "In my professional opinion, releasing the information you request is something that I do not believe will be in the best interests of your client. I am documenting our discussion and that I am telling you this. It will be prominent in the patient's official record." Many times the attorney then says they will think this over and ultimately do not pursue the request. Ultimately, though, it is up to the client to decide if we release the information, even if we recommend against it.

You can also consider adding language to your informed consent agreement such that the client agrees not to call you to testify. This can also be discussed before the client(s) arrive at the first appointment if there is a hint of legal involvement. For example, if being asked to treat a spouse who is divorcing, we routinely have the clients and attorney agree to this request before commencing treatment. This is also true if one wants to try to help insulate and protect the sanctity of the therapeutic treatment environment. Although we may receive a court order for our testimony and records, and we must comply with such an order, having the client agree at the outset that you are providing treatment and not an evaluation, and that you will not testify, may help avoid the piercing of the therapeutic "bubble" of privacy in some circumstances. There are no guarantees, however, such an agreement may serve to help preserve the treatment nature of the professional relationship and not involve the clinician in the client's legal matters.

Build Protections for Unauthorized and Unintended Sharing of Protected Information

With the proliferation of technology, we often have protected information in many different forms and in many different places (i.e., on paper, computers, smart phones, tablets, e-mail, voice mails, faxes, etc.). This allows for many additional avenues of exposure compared to many years ago, when essentially all information was on paper and simply could be locked in a fireproof file cabinet. Also, we can now easily carry this information around with us as we take our smartphones, laptops, or tablets with us when we leave the office.

Just as you should lock your file cabinet, you should also lock your computers, electronic devices, and Internet cloud-based storage areas that may have identifying information. Most of these "locks" are passwords that can be placed on a website, computer device, or smartphone. However, one common mistake is that people select passwords or access codes that are very simple or common (e.g., your name, birthday, a series of numbers, the same code for multiple devices or sites, etc.). Vary these names and codes. Use codes that perhaps only make sense to you and that you can easily remember. For example, the date of a loved one's birthday combined with the backward initials of another loved one and a punctuation mark can be far more difficult for someone to decipher than the numbers "1, 1, 1, 1." Similarly, thumb drives can be purchased that are encrypted and locked, so that if they are lost or stolen your information may be more secure.

You can also encrypt sensitive files that you store in the cloud and on your computer(s). There is free software that will do this for you. Some clinicians encrypt their e-mails to and about clients. When you encrypt a file, anyone who does not have the code for that file will see symbols that do not allow the actual content of the file to be interpreted. When storing information on the cloud, add an easily understood explanation of your data storage and security procedures to your informed consent so your patients are informed of the possible limits of confidentiality (Devereaux & Gottlieb, 2012).

Do not leave old voice mails on your machine. Often voice mails have a four-digit password. If someone works at it, and you have a relatively easy password, they can gain access to your voice mails.

Do not use autodial when sending a fax. If you fax frequently, it is tempting to put common numbers on your fax machine so you do not have to look up the number and dial each time. However, this significantly increases the risk of sending something to the wrong person, as all it takes is pressing one wrong key for the fax to go to a completely different fax machine, so great care and attention to detail are recommended.

Consider not putting last names of your clients in your appointment book or on your electronic device. (At times you may need to use an initial to distinguish between two patients with the same first name.) If your calendar is lost, your patient list will not be immediately identifiable.

Be Prepared for Unexpected Face-to-Face Meetings

In some communities it is quite likely that you will unexpectedly run into clients in public settings (church, social gatherings, school events, athletic events, grocery stores, etc.). These eventualities can be awkward and can lead to breaches, as a friend or child asks you, "Who is that?" Addressing this eventuality in advance, so that you and your patients have an advance agreement on how to handle such situations, can help make for a less awkward moment and avoid an unintended breach.

It is a good idea to discuss with the client(s) what their expectations are should you have an unexpected meeting in public. Many clinicians clarify that they will let the client decide how to handle the situation. That is, they will not initiate contact or recognition unless the client does so first. Also, consider explaining to loved ones that if you meet someone in public who knows you, you may not be able to discuss the context under which you know them.

Communicating by Telephone

At times, a patient you are treating may not have told family members, work colleagues, or roommates they are in counseling. A contact that you initiate to confirm an appointment or to remind a patient about an outstanding balance can cause a breach of the confidentiality that, in some circumstances, can be followed by an acute family disturbance and even domestic violence. Use your informed consent agreement at the outset of treatment to specify what phone numbers you can call. Then, be careful when calling to not use terms like "Doctor" or "therapist" when leaving a message with someone else or on your patient's voice mail. Also, do not assume your patient's voice mail is confidential. It is often best to simply leave your call-back information, even if you are returning a call.

Communicating by US Postal Service

It is important to make sure you have consent to send mail to the patient's residence; otherwise you could be inadvertently violating confidentiality. Many clinicians will stamp all envelopes to patients "Confidential" as a further attempt to preserve confidentiality. Another strategy is to have an ambiguous return address on mail sent to a patient. For example, omitting your name and degree and instead just having your initials (or the initials of your practice) and the street address is a strategy some clinicians use. This is much easier now that you can customize the return address when you print out the envelope.

Communicating by E-mail

E-mail is generally not deemed to be confidential. Although some Internet providers may encrypt transmissions, one's e-mail still can be broken into (hacked), leading to the inadvertent exposure of confidential information. Additionally, if one of your devices that connects to your e-mail is lost, again the potential is there for your e-mails to be exposed, especially if your password is guessed or discovered. We recommend that you develop a policy for e-mail communication. Decide whether you will communicate by e-mail, and whether you will limit the communication to administrative and scheduling issues or also include more personal/clinical matters. These latter topics are riskier from the standpoint of an unintended exposure of confidential information.

You should obtain informed consent regarding the use of e-mail at the start of counseling when the client signs your informed consent agreement. Specify whether or not you will be communicating by e-mail and offer the client the right to decline to receive this form of communication. The agreement should state that you cannot guarantee the confidentiality of e-mails. Additionally, for those clients who desire to communicate in this way, you should review with them the potential risks involved as part of your informed consent discussions. Also, be sure to obtain a personal e-mail address for the client. Corporate or work e-mails are almost never confidential, and you should assume that whatever you communicate with the client may be viewed by the client's employer. In case you accidentally send a client e-mail to the wrong address, you can include a statement with your electronic signature on the bottom of all your e-mails that indicates the message is confidential and requests that any unintended receiver notify you and also destroy any electronic and paper copies.

Consider using a special e-mail service that offers extra encryption. It is important to carefully assess whether the e-mails can be viewed by the personnel at the e-mail provider or are encrypted there as well. You can also assign a separate, complex, and unique password to access your e-mail account to help make it more difficult for someone to access your e-mail if you lose your computing device. Similarly, explore whether your e-mail provider has a two-step authentication process, which potentially can reduce the likelihood of your account being hacked. This process requires you to enter a unique code sent to a different device (e.g., your cell phone) when you are trying to log into your e-mail from an unfamiliar device or location.

Be especially careful when using "Respond to All." You may not have a release to communicate with other people on the distribution list. This is an easy trap to fall into as some of the names in the respond-to-all list may not even be readily visible.

Last, placing a password on each of your devices to help keep them from being accessed in case they are lost or stolen is another step to help protect against the unintended exposure of confidential information. Some devices also have a feature where they can be tracked and disabled if they are lost or stolen. Consider activating this feature.

Seek Input If You Are Not Sure

Rarely is a request for information an emergency. In fact, emergencies are often less of a dilemma, because most of us are trained to forego getting a release in a life-threatening situation. However, in situations where there is not a true emergency, you may still feel pressured by the person requesting the information to jump through hoops and get the information to them immediately. If you accept their anxiety and pressure as your own, you give up the opportunity to carefully assess the request and your options in response. You also forego the option of contacting colleagues and your malpractice carrier to get important input.

It can be useful to have a small network of professionals you trust and who are outside of the immediate situation to provide input and help clarify your action plan in response to the request. This network can also include your malpractice carrier, who may have a professionally staffed help line with senior colleagues to offer guidance and input (not legal advice per se). Writing out your talking points in advance of making a call to respond to a request for information can also be helpful, as it can help you focus and not become distracted by the caller's demands.

SPECIAL SITUATIONS

Thanking Referral Sources

Calling or e-mailing other professionals to thank them for considering you for referrals is typically seen as an important aspect of practice development and maintaining a good working relationship with them. Many clinicians think it is permissible and may not obtain a release, believing they are not disclosing confidential clinical information. However, that client's presence in the office is deemed confidential, and a thank-you call to the referral source can be viewed as a breach if not authorized in advance by the client. It is necessary to get written informed consent from the client in order to contact the referral source.

If you want the referral source to know the patient is scheduled for the first appointment, consider gently informing the patient on the first call that they can notify the referring professional that they have scheduled the appointment. Alternatively, you can discuss the possibility of contacting the referral source when you meet with and talk about confidentiality with the patient. This can also give you the opportunity to clarify whether there are limits to what information the patient wants you to disclose to the referral source. Of course, be sure to obtain written consent to contact the referral source from the client during the first session.

Treating Children and Adolescents

The treatment of children, and especially adolescents, adds another level of complexity when it comes to confidentiality, because there is another party (or parties) who have the rights to waive confidentiality and have their own information protected. These rights can be contrary to what your patient wants and to what you believe is ultimately in your patient's best interests. Ethical complexities can also be increased in families of divorce, where one parent may want the child in psychotherapy and the other does not. The parents may or may not have joint legal custody. If not, one of the parents may have medical decision-making power and deny the other parent the right to information about whether their child is involved in counseling and what is being discussed. Confidentiality rules related to children and adolescents vary by jurisdiction. You should be very informed of the pertinent statues where you practice (relating to age of majority, informing parents, confidentiality, etc.).

In short, know the law. Know what you have to disclose (especially to the child's parents) and at what age it changes. Know whom you need to contact to obtain authority to release information and whether both parents have to provide consent. Be certain who are the legal guardians of your patient. Do not make assumptions that parents are legal guardians. Request to see a copy of the divorce decree if pertinent. Do not simply take one parent's word on this issue. Discuss the limits of confidentiality with the child or adolescent and the parents or guardians at the outset of counseling.

Then, be clear at the outset of treatment what you will and will not disclose to parents or legal guardians. It is often advisable to have part of an early session devoted to this discussion with both the patient and parents present so that a clear understanding is obtained in advance of treatment. Be sure that what you agree to is within the context of the law. For example, a parent may agree to one thing in concept at the beginning of treatment, such as that all discussions with their 10-year-old are confidential. However, if they find they do not like what is taking place in treatment, they may then change their mind and state that by law they are entitled to read their child's file.

Document the agreements around confidentiality, what types of information will not be disclosed to parents, and what information will be disclosed. Remember that if you see the child's siblings or parents, they, too, are likely to be entitled to confidentiality. This will require you to obtain appropriate authorization to release any information that includes mention of their contact with you.

Last, many times other professionals will ask your opinion about family members (children, adolescents, and even the parents) who you may or may not have met, and for whom you almost certainly have not conducted a formal assessment. Providing such information is ill-advised, unwarranted, and additionally inappropriate without informed consent from all parties (the patient and the individual being discussed).

Accepting Cases With Legal Involvement

It is quite common to be asked to be involved in cases where legal issues come into play. Zimmerman, Hess, McGarrah, Benjamin, Ally, Gollan, and Kaiser-Boyd (2009) discuss ethical issues in divorce and child custody issues. They stress the importance of knowing your jurisdiction's laws, avoiding inappropriate advocacy, record-keeping issues, questions to ask in accepting the referral in the first place, countertransference issues, and taking care in communications, among other issues. In addition to divorce cases, your services may be sought around workers' compensation (WC) matters, other civil matters, and even criminal matters. You do not have to be a forensics expert to be sent a referral that seeks your expert testimony. In fact, many psychotherapists are referred patients who are in the midst of litigation as a strategy to better the client's position (e.g., to demonstrate to the court they are working on a problem that led them to court in the first place).

The first step is being certain what your role will be and to whom you are responsible. Are you being hired by the court or by one of the parties? Is your role to be an expert witness or what is termed a "fact witness"? Are you able to do what is asked of you in a way that does not compromise your integrity or the integrity of the professional relationship you have with the people involved? It can be helpful to make it clear from the start whether or not you are willing to take a case in which you may have to testify and under what conditions you are willing to do so. Some clinicians will not engage in treatment with an individual when there is a strong likelihood they will need to testify, as they believe that the treatment itself may be compromised by the outside influence of the client seeking the professional's testimony. Cases in which there has been a personal injury, a domestic situation such as divorce or violence, and WC are situations that hold a high likelihood of the mental health professional being asked to testify.

Additionally, an important issue for early clarification in forensic cases is who will have access to records and reports that may be generated. For example, in a custody case a parental fitness or substance abuse evaluation may serve as a consultation for a guardian ad litem who needs this information to make a better recommendation to the court. In such cases it may be specified that the results are only communicated to them. Neither attorney, nor any member of the divorcing couple, may have access to the report. In other instances the reports are only released to the attorneys and they are prevented from sharing them with their clients. At times the results of the reports may be available to all parties in the divorce. We want to emphasize how important it is to clarify these issues from the outset and to have the agreement in writing signed by all parties. Similarly, it can be helpful to have such evaluations ordered directly by the court. Often clinicians can request this before actually seeing the client. Clinicians who provide parent coordination and co-parent counseling can have their services ordered by the court as well, to obtain clarity regarding confidentiality, the scope of their role, liability, and so forth.

These issues then need to be communicated clearly with the responsible parties to make sure you indeed have informed consent. Imagine being in the position as the psychotherapist of a 12 year-old whose parents are divorcing. The child tells you information about his father's anger that, when you testify, weighs heavily against the father's attempts to secure custody. The child not only feels the confidentiality of the treatment has been breached, but also has to deal with his father's rage for "being thrown under the bus." This could have been avoided if your role and reporting responsibilities were clear to all from the start, and if limits had been set about whether or not you would testify. In active litigation, before you accept the referral, you can actually ask for orders from the court or a written agreement signed by the attorneys that outlines your role and whether or not you will be testifying. You also can specify what conditions you require in order to begin working on the case. A client being court-ordered to see you does not mean that you are court-ordered to see the client under all conditions and circumstances. We have worked through referring attorneys to get orders rewritten so that they are acceptable for the services being provided.

It can be helpful to ask the referral source or caller (before the prospective client arrives) if there is active litigation and what the intent is related to the referral. When doing so you can try to assess whether the prospect of your testimony will compromise any treatment being considered as a result of the release of the client's confidential information, and the pressing need the client has for you to provide favorable testimony. It is important to be absolutely clear about whether you are functioning in an evaluative role for the court or in a treatment role.

At the outset of your professional relationship, clearly establish the limits of confidentiality and the risks associated with your potential testimony. It is important to specify how your testimony might not ultimately be in the client's best interests and might jeopardize the psychotherapeutic relationship. Make sure your written and signed informed consent to treatment specifies your relationship to the client and the limits to confidentiality.

Referrals by Employers or Schools

Employers and schools often directly seek the services of mental health professionals. Employers may call on you to see a client in an employee assistance program, provide a substance abuse evaluation, assess fitness for duty, provide a critical-incident debriefing, or offer executive coaching. Schools may ask you to see staff as well as students for similar reasons, or to treat and assess students who they are concerned may be at risk of injury to self or others or may be affected by significant emotional issues. It is likely that the employer or school, as well as the employee, student, or parent(s), will not understand or have not discussed the complexities of the ethical dilemma posed by the referral. For example, if the school or employer is paying for your services, it is crucial to determine and be clear with the person(s) to whom you are providing services exactly who the client actually is (i.e., the school/employer or the employee/student's legal guardian) and what the expectations will be regarding your role and confidentiality.

Just as in other circumstances, when dealing with schools and employers you should clearly discuss your role and obligations to the employer/school with the client/legal guardian at the start of your first appointment. The client/legal guardian should sign an informed consent form that clearly specifies your relationship with the employer or school and any limitations around confidentiality. At times, the individual being evaluated is not actually the client and will not have access to the results of the evaluation, as they will be released to "the client" (e.g., the school or employer). Thus, these issues should be clarified from the outset.

You should make sure your billing office knows who to submit the bill to and whether or not the client's name should appear on the bill. Often, when billing the school/employer, the client's name should not appear on the bill (to protect the client's confidentiality). The word "consultation" without the employee's name may be enough for a bill that you submit to the employer or the school. If they require more, you can come up with a simple coding system that protects confidentiality of your client by not putting identifying information on the bill but allows your contact at the organization to know to whom you rendered services.

Workers' Compensation

Most of the focus on job-related injuries is placed on physical illness. However, physical injuries can have an emotional component that (a) is a result of the injury or (b) makes it more difficult to recover from the physical injury. Walfish (2006) points out that WC policies and procedures have been created by statute and vary from state to state. Therefore, it is imperative that if a clinician is going to see an injured worker, prior to doing so they need to learn about documentation requirements and the rules about confidentiality.

Most WC policies actually provide no confidentiality for the injured worker. Clinical records often need to be included in order for payment to be received for sessions. Discussions may take place between the clinician and a case manager about the injured worker and their clinical needs and progress. However, the case manager may be employed by the state, a rehabilitation company, or some other third party involved in the WC system. Psychological evaluations and psychotherapy treatment records may be considered part of an "open system," in that the individuals paying for services or benefits to the injured worker are provided access to these documents. As such it is imperative that clients choosing to participate in treatment understand that they are basically waiving their right to confidentiality when they choose to participate in the WC system. Further, if the case is litigated, then the clinician likely will be asked to testify about their psychotherapeutic work in a forensic setting, and no information related to the evaluation or treatment provided can be considered confidential. It is up to us to clearly explain this to the client, as we cannot be sure the other professionals in the case have done so.

Dealing With the Media

Mental health clinicians are sometimes contacted by members of the media requesting comments on timely issues and topics relevant to the professional's areas of expertise. For example, when a mass shooting is in the news, the observations, comments, and insights of a mental health professional may be sought.

When contacted by the media, there is often urgency due to the pressures of a deadline. Additional pressure may result from the emotional content, timeliness, and seriousness of the story. An ego or prestige factor also may be at play, depending on who is seeking your input. All of these factors can lead to ethical problems, both in terms of confidentiality and the possible exploitation of your patients.

Often, members of the media will not only ask for your professional opinions about a particular event or issue, but they also will ask for clinical examples from your practice or for you to refer them to some of your clients so they can be interviewed as well. For example, the media may be doing a story about the suicide of a high-profile person. Although it would be very appropriate to share general information about depression, suicide, suicide prevention, and treatment if these are your areas of expertise, it would not be appropriate to speculate on the individual in question or to share information about any of the clients you are treating who may be struggling with these issues. The interviewer may request names and contact information of clients who struggled with depression and suicide who are "success stories" to interview. The interviewer may even stress to you all the good this will do in providing needed education about these important issues to the public. Regardless, you should only provide general information and you should never violate your clients' confidentiality or act in ways that are not consistent with their best interests. For further information on and discussion of ethics issues and dilemmas related to interactions with the media, see McGarrah, Alvord, Martin, and Haldeman (2009).

Dealing With Collections Agencies

By the time you start to deal with a collections agency, you may be emotional about the situation. It is easy to lose perspective, especially if you feel the patient literally stole from you. That is, they stole your time and your investment in the psychotherapeutic process, and then ignored your own attempts at collection of the agreed-upon fees, which perhaps further frustrated you. Now it seems you are left with no choice but to "send them to collections." This is a risky time for you and your practice. Your own emotions (or countertransference) are high and the likelihood of a grievance against your license is also high, should you pursue collections (Bennett, Bricklin, Harris, Knapp, VandeCreek, & Younggren, 2006). It can be especially problematic if you try to exact retribution from a responsible party by withholding a request for records due to the client having an outstanding balance.

From a practice management perspective, the problem of having a high outstanding balance is a problem in the way accounts receivables are addressed. The need to retain a collections agency should be avoided by having policies, procedures, and safeguards established to avoid being in the situation in the first place. Although this is not within the scope of this book, Walfish and Barnett (2009) address this at length.

The question of being sensitive to the ethical issues, though, is important when it comes to collections. Perhaps the two most important concepts have to do with notice to the responsible party that you are pursuing collections and taking great care about the information you send to the collections agency. Be sure to have the agency sign a HIPAA Business Associates Contract. See the website of the US Department of Health & Human Services at http://www.hhs.gov/ocr/privacy/hipaa/understanding/coveredentities/contractprov.html for Sample Business Associate Contract Provisions. Put a notice in your informed consent agreement that you reserve the right to use a collections agency to aid in collecting uncollected fees.

Before referring the case to the collections agency, give the patient written notice of this possibility and time to resolve the financial issue. Your jurisdiction may have specific regulations as to what must occur (e.g., the number of attempts, types of attempts, and time frames associated with the pursuit of collections) before you can turn the account over to collections.

Try to personally contact the patient to see what the problem is and whether it is possible to negotiate some sort of settlement agreeable to you both. For example, it might be useful to hear that the patient did not show or pay for the last appointment because they felt slighted by you in some way (e.g., kept them waiting, answered an emergency call in their session, was not professional in some way, etc.). A direct call between you and the patient (not from your office manager) can give you a chance to address the matter, rather than have it escalate into a claim to the licensing board.

If sending information to a collections agency, only share the patient's name and address, date of service, fee charged, and amount owed. Never share clinical information such as their diagnosis. It is important to make sure that your billing staff knows this as well. Sending copies of what was submitted to insurance or discussing the clinical status of the patient with the collections agency is not appropriate.

In summary, there are many things you can do to decrease the risk of inadvertent communication of confidential or protected information. The obligation is not to prevent every possible occurrence, but rather to employ safeguards to avoid foreseeable breaches. That is, a burglar can break into your office in the middle of the night and ransack your files. It is not expected that you will have guard dogs, laser alarms, and other Fort Knox setups to foil the intruder. It is expected, though, that you will lock your files, not leave an easily accessible key, and lock your office door. The expectation is that you will do what you reasonably can to protect your patients' confidentiality. This level of reasonable action changes over time as technology changes and also based on the type and size of your practice. Larger organizations are expected to have more advanced security measures in place. As technology has evolved, it is now easier for someone in solo practice to have some of those same protections (e.g., encrypted files) at little or no cost.

ETHICAL CHALLENGES

- It can be difficult to distinguish between one's ethical obligations around confidentiality and the demands of a legal or social situation.
- It can be confusing as to who has the right to release information and who is covered by confidentiality statutes.

- We can miss subtle ethical requirements by virtue of our involvement in an ethically demanding situation.
- Knowing how to respond to requests for records and clinical information in emotionally charged situations.
- Determining who the client is, and thus who has the right to have access to confidential information, and who has the right to authorize the release of confidential information.

KEY POINTS TO KEEP IN MIND

- It is important to protect against foreseeable violations of the protection of health-related information and confidentiality.
- Anticipation, preparation, and obtaining informed consent in advance of disclosure is a good practice.
- Be sure there is clarity in advance about who and what will be released and how the information will be used.
- Documentation of discussions about confidentiality and related agreements is essential.

PRACTICAL RECOMMENDATIONS

- Establish routine policies and procedures that help protect confidentiality and limit the likelihood of accidental mishaps.
- Be clear about the limits of confidentiality in your informed consent document.
- Keep up with your professional association newsletters and listservs, as they often have discussions of technological advances that can help protect health information.
- Seek input when you are not sure or feel pressured to release information.
- Be sure to provide a thorough informed consent to all responsible parties, clarifying the limits of confidentiality, to whom you will be releasing information, and the possible ramifications of such a release.

PITFALLS TO AVOID

- Reacting quickly when stressed by time or outside pressure to communicate information.
- Not establishing protocols and procedures to handle routine requests.
- Not seeking input from colleagues.
- Assuming that a signed release means that informed consent is in place.

- Assuming you only need one signature from parents, especially if they are separated or divorced.
- Assuming a given parent is the legal guardian in a divorce.
- Taking a less than serious approach about securing unwarranted access to confidential protected information.

RELEVANT ETHICS CODE STANDARDS

Third-Party Services and Requests for Information

- AAMFT Code of Ethics (AAMFT, 2012) Principle 1.13, Relationships With Third Parties, states, "Marriage and family therapists, upon agreeing to provide services to a person or entity at the request of a third party, clarify to the extent feasible, and at the outset of the service, the nature of the relationship with each party and the limits of confidentiality" (p. 3).
- ACA Code of Ethics (ACA, 2005) Standard B.2.c., Court-Ordered Disclosure, states, "When subpoenaed to release confidential or privileged information without a client's permission, counselors obtain written, informed consent from the client or take steps to prohibit the disclosure or have it limited as narrowly as possible due to potential harm to the client or counseling relationship" (p. 7).
- APA Ethics Code (APA, 2010) Standard 3.11, Psychological Services Delivered to or Through Organizations, states that psychologists "provide information beforehand to clients and when appropriate those directly affected by the services about (1) the nature and objectives of the services, (2) the intended recipients, (3) which of the individuals are clients, (4) the relationship the psychologist will have with each person and the organization, (5) the probable uses of services provided and information obtained, (6) who will have access to the information, and (7) limits of confidentiality" (p. 6).
- NASW Code of Ethics (NASW, 2008) Standard 1.07j, Privacy and Confidentiality, states, "Social workers should protect the confidentiality of clients during legal proceedings to the extent permitted by law. When a court of law or other legally authorized body orders social workers to disclose confidential or privileged information without a client's consent and such disclosure could cause harm to the client, social workers should request that the court withdraw the order or limit the order as narrowly as possible or maintain the records under seal, unavailable for public inspection" (p. 3).

Public Disclosures and the Media

- AAMFT Code of Ethics (AAMFT, 2012) Principle 3.13, Public Statements, states, "Marriage and family therapists, because of their ability to influence and alter the lives of others, exercise special care when making public their recommendations and opinions through testimony and other public statements" (p. 4).

- ACA Code of Ethics (ACA, 2005) Standard B.1.b., Respect for Privacy, states, "Counselors respect client rights to privacy. Counselors solicit private information from clients only when it is beneficial to the counseling process" (p. 7). Further, Standard B.1.c., Respect for Confidentiality, states, "Counselors do not share confidential information without client consent or without sound legal or ethical justification" (p. 7).
- APA Ethics Code (APA, 2010) Standard 5.04, Media Presentations, states, "When psychologists provide public advice or comment via print, Internet or other electronic transmission, they take precautions to ensure that statements (1) are based on their professional knowledge, training or experience in accord with appropriate psychological literature and practice; (2) are otherwise consistent with this Ethics Code; and (3) do not indicate that a professional relationship has been established with the recipient" (p. 8).
- NASW Code of Ethics (NASW, 2008) Standard 1.07k, Privacy and Confidentiality, states "Social workers should protect the confidentiality of clients when responding to requests from members of the media" (p. 3).

Fees and Collections

- AAMFT Code of Ethics (AAMFT, 2012) Principle 7, Financial Arrangements, states, "Marriage and family therapists make financial arrangements with clients, third-party payors, and supervisees that are reasonably understandable and conform to accepted professional practices" (p. 7).
- ACA Code of Ethics (ACA, 2005) Standard A.10.C., Nonpayment of Fees, states, "If counselors intend to use collection agencies or take legal measures to collect fees from clients who do not pay for services as agreed upon, they first inform clients of intended actions and offer clients the opportunity to make payment" (p. 6).
- APA Ethics Code (APA, 2010) Standard 6.04a, Fees and Financial Arrangements, states, "As early as is feasible in a professional or scientific relationship, psychologists and recipients of psychological services reach an agreement specifying compensation and billing arrangements" (p. 9).
- NASW Code of Ethics (NASW, 2008) Standard 1.13a, Payment for Services, states, "When setting fees, social workers should ensure that the fees are fair, reasonable, and commensurate with the services performed. Consideration should be given to clients' ability to pay" (p. 4).

Using Technology in Practice

- AAMFT Code of Ethics (AAMFT, 2012) Principle 1.14, Electronic Therapy, states, "Prior to commencing therapy services through electronic means (including but not limited to phone and internet), marriage and family therapists ensure that they are compliant with all relevant laws for the delivery of such services" (p. 3).
- ACA Code of Ethics (ACA, 2005) Standard B.3.e., Transmitting Confidential Information, states, "Counselors take precautions to ensure the confidentiality of information transmitted through the use of computers, electronic mail, facsimile machines, telephones, voicemail, answering machines, and other electronic or computer technology" (p. 8).
- APA Ethics Code (APA, 2010) Standard 4.01, Maintaining Confidentiality, states, "Psychologists have a primary obligation and take reasonable precautions to protect confidential information obtained through or stored in any medium, recognizing that the extent and limits of confidentiality may be regulated by law or established by institutional rules or professional or scientific relationship" (p. 7).
- NASW Code of Ethics (NASW, 2008) Standard 1.07l, Privacy and Confidentiality, states, "Social workers should protect the confidentiality of clients' written and electronic records and other sensitive information. Social workers should take reasonable steps to ensure that clients' records are stored in a secure location and that clients' records are not available to others who are not authorized to have access" (p. 3). Additionally, Standard 1.07m states, "Social workers should take precautions to ensure and maintain the confidentiality of information transmitted to other parties through the use of computers, electronic mail, facsimile machines, telephones and telephone answering machines, and other electronic or computer technology. Disclosure of identifying information should be avoided whenever possible" (p. 3).

Confidentiality and Informed Consent

- AAMFT Code of Ethics (AAMFT, 2012) Principle 2.2, Written Authorization to Release Client Information, states, "Marriage and family therapists do not disclose client confidences except by written authorization or wavier, or where mandated or permitted by law" (p. 3).
- ACA Code of Ethics (ACA, 2005) Standard B.2.d., Minimal Disclosure, states, "To the extent possible, clients are informed before confidential information is disclosed and are involved in the disclosure decision-making process. When circumstances require the disclosure of confidential information, only essential information is revealed" (p. 7).

- APA Ethics Code (APA, 2010) Standard 10.01a, Informed Consent to Therapy, states that "psychologists inform clients/patients as early as is feasible in the therapeutic relationship about the nature and anticipated course of therapy, fees, involvement of third parties and limits of confidentiality" (p. 13).
- NASW Code of Ethics (NASW, 2008) Standard 1.07b, Privacy and Confidentiality, states, "Social workers may disclose confidential information when appropriate with valid consent from a client or a person legally authorized to consent on behalf of a client" (p. 3).

REFERENCES

American Association for Marriage and Family Therapy. (2012). *Code of ethics*. Retrieved from http://www.aamft.org/imis15/content/legal_ethics/code_of_ethics.aspx

American Counseling Association. (2005). *ACA code of ethics*. Retrieved from http://www.counseling.org/Resources/aca-code-of-ethics.pdf

American Psychological Association. (2010). *Ethical principles of psychologists and code of conduct*. Retrieved from http://www.apa.org/ethics

Bennett, B. E., Bricklin, P. M., Harris, E., Knapp, S., VandeCreek, L., & Younggren, J. N. (2006). *Assessing and managing risk in psychological practice: An individualized approach*. Rockville, MD: The Trust.

Devereaux, R. L., & Gottlieb, M. C. (2012). Record keeping in the cloud: Ethical considerations. *Professional Psychology: Research and Practice, 43*, 627–632. doi:10.1037/a0028268

McGarrah, N. A., Alvord, M. K., Martin, J. N., & Haldeman, D. C. (2009). In the public eye: The ethical practice of media psychology. *Professional Psychology: Research and Practice, 40*, 172–180.

National Association of Social Workers. (2008). *Code of ethics*. Retrieved from http://www.socialworkers.org/pubs/code/code.asp

U.S. Department of Health and Human Services. (1996). Health Insurance Portability and Accountability Act of 1996. Retrieved from http://www.hhs.gov/ocr/privacy/

Walfish, S. (2006). Conducting personal injury evaluations. In I. Weiner & A. K. Hess (Eds.), *Handbook of forensic psychology* (3rd ed., pp. 124–139). New York, NY: Wiley.

Walfish, S., & Barnett, J. E., (2009). *Financial success in mental health practice: Essential tools and strategies for practitioners*. Washington, DC: APA Books.

Zimmerman, J., Hess, A. K., McGarrah, N. A., Benjamin, G. A., Ally, G. A., Gollan, J. K., & Kaiser-Boyd, N. (2009). Ethical and professional considerations in divorce and child custody cases. *Professional Psychology: Research and Practice, 40*, 539–549.

RELEASE OF INFORMATION CHECKLIST
(All items must be checked)

☐ There is a valid signed release on file that specifies to whom the information is to be released, the purpose of the release, and what specific information is being requested.

☐ The relationship of the person seeking the information to the patient is clearly known.

☐ The patient(s) or responsible individual(s) have been contacted by the clinician and informed about the request and the possible negative consequences of releasing the information, and still consent to the release.

☐ The patient's clinician has examined the file to make sure there is not information in the file that would be inappropriate to release (e.g., misfiled information from a different case, information that would be psychologically damaging to the patient, information that was from other sources, etc.).

☐ The content of the file is in order (e.g., sorted by date).

☐ There have been no alternations to the content of the file.

☐ Any allowed charges for copying of a file have been posted to the patient's account or billed to the person requesting the information.

☐ If the patient is to receive or have access to the information in the file, every attempt has been made to schedule an opportunity for the patient to review the file with his/her clinician and the clinician has checked the file to make sure there is not information included that, if released, would be harmful to the patient.

☐ Only a copy (not the original) of the file is being released.

5

Financial Decisions

Charging fees for providing mental health services and collecting those fees are issues that almost everyone who has chosen to go into private practice has faced. After all, most individuals enter this field "to help others" and often this sense of altruism can come into conflict with having to charge and collect fees for the services we provide. This may be especially true when we perceive that paying for our services may be a financial hardship for a client.

Walfish and Barnett's (2009) First Principle of Private Practice Success states, "You need to resolve the conflict between altruism and being a business owner" (p. 8). If this conflict is not resolved, the private practitioner may become vulnerable to making clinical and business errors and engaging in unethical behaviors. These may occur even when the clinician has the best of intentions and is motivated by a desire to help their client. This is borne out by Barnett and Johnson's (2008) statement: "Conflicts and misunderstandings related to fees and financial arrangements constitute one of the most frequent and preventable sources of legal and ethical complaints against psychologists" (p. 106). Bennett, Bricklin, Harris, Knapp, VandeCreek, and Younggren (2006) present data to support this statement. In reviewing disciplinary actions by the APA Ethics Committee for a 10-year period, they found that insurance and fee problems tied (with nonsexual multiple relationship issues) for the second most frequent category of complaints made against psychologists, superseded only by sexual misconduct.

Barnett and Walfish (2011) suggest that billing and collecting fees should be an easy and straightforward process. The informed consent agreement that has been presented to the client, reviewed with the client, and agreed upon with the client serves as a contract for payment of fees for services provided. However, Barnett and Walfish note there may be resistance from the client and/or the clinician to carrying out this straightforward process. They suggest that resistance from the client may be related to transference issues, such as feelings of entitlement, a discomfort or dislike for "paying for help," or an unwillingness to admit they cannot afford fees for psychotherapy. They also suggest that clinician resistance may be due to a lack of training in business (it is the exception rather than the rule that business of practice issues are discussed during graduate training) or countertransference issues, such as (a) not having resolved the conflict between altruism and being a small business owner (possibly resulting in the buildup of a large balance due), (b) "colluding" with a client against their managed care company (MCO) to get the insurer to pay for uncovered services, or (c) being fearful of having the client become angry at them (and therefore not reasonably enforcing no-show or late cancelation policies).

The key to reducing ethical transgressions is to include all financial issues in the Informed Consent for Treatment Agreement that the client receives upon entering treatment, and to openly discuss and review this document with each client as part of the informed consent process. This document serves as a financial contract between the client and the private practitioner. It fosters autonomy in client decision making about entering or remaining in psychotherapy with a particular clinician. Additionally, by providing full disclosure of the costs of services and the procedures for collecting fees from the outset, the client and psychotherapist may hold each other accountable regarding their agreement on the financial aspects of their relationship. At the very least, the informed consent agreement should include information regarding (a) the fee charged for each service provided; (b) whether insurance is accepted or the psychotherapist is an out-of-network provider; (c) when payment is expected; (d) what forms of payment are accepted (e.g., cash, check, credit card); (e) what will occur if an outstanding balance accrues; (f) fees charged for late cancelations or missed appointments; (g) fees due, if any, for additional report writing or completing of forms (e.g., disability insurance or life insurance); (h) fees due, if any, for telephone calls or e-mails between sessions; (i) fees charged for forensic services, including consultation with attorneys, review of records to prepare for testimony, testimony in deposition or court, and travel time to and from court; and (j) a statement about whether fee increases are anticipated and how these will be handled.

Financial issues, and the ethical issues that emerge from them, should be at the forefront of private practitioners' minds if they are to be successful both clinically and in business. The issues are plentiful and complicated and have been the focus of our previous writings in an entire book (Barnett & Walfish, 2011). In this chapter we address several of the most salient issues, including (a) setting of fees, (b) sliding scale arrangements, (c) increasing fees, (d) collections actions, (e) insurance issues, (f) informing clients of the nature and limits of their insurance coverage, (g) accurate billing, (h) what information is to be shared with a MCO, and (i) how to respond if an MCO denies payment for care.

FEE SETTING PRACTICES

The ethics codes of each of the mental health professions highlight the importance of fee arrangements in the delivery of mental health services. Thus it is important that all mental health professionals thoughtfully attend to the ethical implications of financial arrangements made with clients.

Fee setting is easy if you have signed a contract with an insurance carrier agreeing to see their subscribers. There are no ethical issues to be grappled with as the fees are set by contractual arrangement. If you are a Blue Cross/Blue Shield provider in State X, you have agreed to a specific fee for each of your services. For example, this may be $80.00 for a 45-minute session of psychotherapy (CPT Code 90834). This means that although your usual and customary fee may be $160.00 for this service, you are only entitled to receive a total of $80.00, due to the contractual arrangement. Note that it can be illegal (and thus unethical) and against the contract you have signed to "balance bill" for this service. That is, it is not ethical to tell the client they are also responsible for the additional $80.00 not paid by the combination of the copayment and the insurer's payment so that you can collect your usual and customary fee of $160.00.

Fee setting outside of insurance is more complicated because each individual clinician must choose the amount they will charge. This figure may be influenced by the economy in your local area, specialized services you offer, the amount of competition in the area from other private practitioners, number of years in practice, the client's ability to pay for services, and your emotional comfort with money. Walfish and Barnett's (2009) 12th Principle of Private Practice Success states, "Clinicians should charge fees that the market will bear. To charge less does not make good business sense. To charge more does not make good business sense" (p. 119). Working in a free-market economy, clinicians are free to charge whatever fees they would like, and it is up to potential clients to determine if they want to purchase these services at the price being charged. However, from an ethics perspective there is an exception for the private practitioner to consider. First, the clinician cannot exert "undue influence" over clients in setting their fees. For example, because the client may be in emotional pain and in a "vulnerable position" by seeking out services in the first place, the clinician cannot take advantage of this by charging outrageous fees. So, if the community standard is $100 per session, clinicians may be seen as exerting undue influence if they charge $500 per session. This may be viewed as taking advantage of someone in a vulnerable position for personal gain. Raising fees significantly without notice for vulnerable clients would be another example of exerting undue influence solely for the purpose of personal gain by the clinician.

The fee charged may be part of the consideration leading a client to choose to work with Private Practitioner A versus Private Practitioner B. Clients may have a certain fee in mind they feel is appropriate and are comfortable paying for psychotherapy services. They may want to budget only a certain percentage of their income or savings in seeking out these services. This is an autonomous choice by the client. As noted, practitioners must let the client know as early as feasible the costs of services. Many clinicians list their fees on their websites. Many clinicians will discuss fees in the initial telephone call when arranging the appointment. What would be suboptimal, from both a clinical and business of practice perspective, would be to have a client come in for an initial intake, spend 55 minutes "pouring their hearts out" and developing a therapeutic alliance with an empathic and intuitive clinician, and then find out in the last 5 minutes of the session that the psychotherapy fee they were hoping to pay was only 50% of what the actual cost would be for them to continue in treatment. Informing clients of fees charged after they have already become engaged in a treatment process is contradictory to our obligations to clients. If this information is not placed on the website or discussed during the initial telephone call, a careful review of fees in the informed consent agreement at the beginning of an intake session is an essential first step.

Fee setting should not only take into consideration the client's ability to pay for treatment, but should also be dictated by the clinical needs of the client. This is borne out in several ways. First, during the initial intake session you should develop a general idea of how long the person may be in counseling. Of course it is impossible to predict an exact number of sessions, and it is impossible to predict issues that may arise during the course of counseling that might increase the duration of treatment. However, this general idea should then be matched to the client's ability to pay for treatment. This ability may include amount of insurance coverage available. Some policies have limits on number of sessions per year or lifetime amount spent. Although parity legislation (i.e., coverage for mental health treatment is treated the same as coverage for physical illnesses) does address some of the past discrimination by insurance policies, there are so many exceptions to this rule (e.g., self-insured vs. group policies, biologically based diagnoses vs. adjustment disorders) that it cannot be counted upon. Thus, it is essential that clinicians become aware (either directly on their own or through their client) of the coverage that is available to pay for treatment. For example, if coverage is limited to 20 sessions per year, you should not take on a client who is looking for personality restructuring or psychoanalysis, if additional funds are not available for the client to complete the treatment being sought.

The second way the clinical needs of the client are borne out in the setting of fees is in the determination of needed frequency of sessions during the treatment planning process. In developing their diagnosis and subsequent treatment plan, clinicians should determine the clinically appropriate frequency of sessions. Based on their clinical presentation, does this person need to be seen weekly, twice weekly, every other week, or monthly, and in certain crisis situations do they need to be seen daily? Once this is determined, an assessment can be made as to whether the client can afford the recommended counseling. If not, then either a reduced fee must be offered (see the Sliding Fee Scale Arrangements section, next), or alternative treatment arrangements made to accommodate the client's ability to follow the recommended treatment plan. These alternative arrangements may include a referral to a publicly funded mental health agency (e.g., community mental health center), a nonprofit agency that provides mental health treatment (e.g., family service agencies; a denominationally funded agency such as Jewish Family Services or Catholic Charities), or a university training clinic. It is not prudent for a private practitioner to make a clinical determination that a client needs to be seen weekly for counseling, but chooses only to see them monthly because "that's all the client could afford." Such a plan is not in the client's best interests.

The third way the clinical needs of the client are borne out in the setting of fees is in the choice of treatment modality. The treatment planning process should identify the problem areas to be addressed in counseling as well as the best modality for addressing these specific problems. For example, clinicians may offer both individual and group psychotherapy in their practice. If, in the treatment planning process, individual treatment is identified as the best modality to address a client's particular issues, then treatment must be conducted on an individual basis. Group psychotherapy is less expensive per hour than individual psychotherapy, but this should be selected based on the client's clinical needs, not solely because it is "more affordable." When clients' treatment needs and affordable services offered do not match, an appropriate referral should be made so that the client's best interests are served.

SLIDING FEE SCALE ARRANGEMENTS

Contrary to a stereotype, by and large, private practitioners are not "just in it for the money." From a humanistic point of view private practitioners realize that not all clients can afford their full or standard fee. Indeed, in an effort to balance altruism with the need to run a successful small business, Martin-Causey (2005) describes devoting 10% to 20% of her time to seeing lower fee clients.

There is no right or wrong amount by which to reduce fees. One may work this out on an individual basis or just set a low fee (e.g., $40 or $25 or $10) for a certain number of psychotherapy slots that fit your comfort level. However, when you do reduce your fee, it is important to document this in the client's record along with the reason why you are doing so. In addition, it is important to have the client sign an agreement that, should there be a change in their financial status at a later date, this fee may be renegotiated upward.

It is important to note that one cannot reduce their fee when a client has insurance and the clinician is a participating provider for that carrier. The insurance carrier expects you to charge the contractually agreed-upon fee and to collect the copay and deductible that are due. Further, it may also be illegal to routinely waive copays or deductibles for your clients and this is likely to be seen as a violation of your contract with the insurer. Routinely waiving deductibles and copayments may also create a competitive advantage over clinicians who follow their contract and do not waive their copay. It will be natural for clients to prefer and seek out the services of mental health professionals who waive copays and deductibles, because this results in them paying less for treatment. Again, such a practice is usually a violation of one's contracts with the insurance companies and may result in adverse legal consequences.

This does not mean that copays can never be waived for hardship reasons. Medicare regulations (http://oig.hhs.gov/fraud/docs/alertsandbulletins/121994.html) indicate that copays can be forgiven on an occasional basis. If a fee is being waived it is important to document in the client's treatment record a rationale for why this is being done. However, it could be considered fraudulent if done on a routine basis.

INCREASING FEES

Private practitioners do not have an annual performance review with a supervisor where, if they are deemed to have exceeded expectations in their work, they receive a raise in their salary, in addition to a standard cost of living adjustment. Besides reducing overhead expenses or developing a better paying product line, the only way for private practitioners to receive a raise is to increase their fees.

There is nothing unethical about raising fees per se. Rather, the important issue from an ethics perspective is how and when clients are informed that a fee increase may occur. If the clinician ever intends to raise their fees, it is essential that they indicate that this possibility might occur in the initial informed consent agreement. When these increases may occur and by what percentage should be explicitly spelled out to the client in this document. For example, it may state that fees will rise on the first of January each year by $15.00 or by 5%. By providing this information clients can make a fully informed autonomous decision about how much money they may be spending on psychotherapy services. This is likely not going to be an issue for someone who plans on being in counseling for a brief time (e.g., 6–10 sessions). However, it may be a significant issue for someone who plans on being in counseling for two to three years (or more).

If clients are not forewarned that fees may increase, it may be argued that they were not provided with full disclosure of financial arrangements for the psychotherapy they are seeking and have contracted for with their clinician. Additionally, if a client begins treatment at one fee, shares his or her story, becomes emotionally vulnerable with and possibly even becomes dependent on the clinician, and then the clinician abruptly increases the fee significantly and without adequate notice, this will likely be seen as exploitative of the client. If the client has developed a strong therapeutic alliance with the psychotherapist (though an unexpected fee increase might cause a rupture in this alliance that would need to be addressed), he or she may be reluctant to leave treatment, find a new psychotherapist, and "start all over." Those clients who can't afford the significant fee increase may choose to cease being in counseling. In addition to informing clients of possible fee increases from the outset, it is vital that mental health clinicians provide clients with sufficient notice of impending fee increases so they may be discussed and processed openly in treatment, alternative arrangements to include referrals can be made if needed, and no advantage is taken of the client.

COLLECTIONS

Mental health clinicians who are not comfortable with the business aspects of private practice may experience difficulties collecting fees from their clients. When this occurs it is not unusual for ethical transgressions to follow as a consequence of this discomfort.

Barnett and Walfish (2011) have recommended that the informed consent agreement clearly articulate the specific responsibilities that clients have in paying their fees. Clients should know that if health insurance is being utilized to help pay for treatment, then the client is responsible for paying the portion of any deductible that may be due for the year, plus the copay due for the session. If insurance is not being utilized, the client is responsible to pay the agreed-upon fee. Woody (1988) advises that one way to prevent malpractice is to not allow clients to accrue a deficit in payments. In their sample Informed Consent Agreement, Barnett and Walfish suggest the following example regarding unpaid balances: "Dr. Public will not allow a balance to build up to more than $300, except in the case of a life-threatening emergency" (p. 106). Clients are also informed that discussion will take place regarding the unpaid balance of the bill (once again, note the need for clinicians to feel comfortable with the "business of practice") and that arrangements will be made for payment of the balance or alternative treatment arrangements will be recommended, taking into consideration the client's clinical needs.

The prudent practitioner will make sure that appropriate fees are collected on the day services are provided. There are times when clients do indeed forget their checkbooks. They should be reminded to mail in their overdue payment prior to the next scheduled session, or just bring the payment to the next meeting. To prevent a buildup of a large balance, Barnett and Walfish (2011) also suggest accepting payment by credit card. They present a sample Credit Card Guaranty of Payment form that can be included in the initial intake paperwork. With this form the client is providing permission to the private practitioner to charge their credit card for any unpaid balances after a certain period of time. Although this is not a foolproof method (e.g. at times credit cards are rejected due to having reached their available limit, or their numbers are written down incorrectly), we have found this reduces the likelihood of a large balance being built up. The key is to be proactive and not let the balance get out of hand in the first place.

There is no ethical mandate that states that clinicians must continue to see a client for counseling if the client is not living up to the agreed-upon financial contract. Clinicians may appropriately refer for more affordable treatment if they are not being paid. Although clients may feel "psychologically abandoned" or betrayed, this is (a) a transference reaction, and (b) not considered professional abandonment. Younggren and Gottlieb (2008) point out that the

> psychotherapist's duty does not stop when money or benefits run out, and the psychotherapist still has a fiduciary responsibility to assist, stabilize, and/ or refer patients who are in crisis. However, this does not obligate the psychotherapist to provide extensive pro bono services. (p. 501)

COLLECTION ACTIONS

As with any small business owner, if client fees are not paid the private practitioner can enlist the aid of a collection agency or file an action in small claims court. There is no ethical restriction against taking such actions, as the client has violated their portion of the contract by not living up to their agreed-upon financial obligations.

There are two caveats to the private practitioner taking these actions. The first is ethical (giving the client adequate notice), and the second is practical (assessing the cost/benefit of such action). We have known clinicians who, upon learning of an unpaid balance due from a client, have written a letter stating, "Please bring this balance due to zero within 30 days. If this amount is not paid within 30 days we will be forced to turn your account over to a collection agency." In our opinion, this is not adequate notice. Rather, we advocate for placing this information in the initial informed consent agreement. In this way a client knows from the beginning of treatment that this is a possibility if balances due are unpaid. It may be that the client would choose not to work with a clinician who might have such a policy in place. If they knew this, they may have chosen to work with another practitioner who, rightly or wrongly, they do not perceive as "only being about the money." If a psychologist does choose to turn over an account to a collection agency, Bennett et al. (2006) note the importance of only sharing the minimal information necessary to collect on the claim and not providing any clinical information. Clinicians also need to remember that if they contract with an agency to collect fees on their behalf, the clinician is responsible for the behavior of their agent. Therefore, if the collection agency engages in unscrupulous actions in an attempt to collect funds, or inadvertently violates confidentiality, the clinician may be held accountable. Additionally, state statute may also dictate what actions need to be taken in advance of proceeding to each of the steps in the collection process and whether or not you may charge interest against an unpaid balance.

The second caveat to consider is whether there is wisdom in taking such collection actions. The wisdom has two components. First, on a practical basis how much money will the clinician actually recoup if they pursue this avenue? For example, let's imagine that the clinician has mistakenly allowed a balance to accrue of $500. Although this is the amount due, you will have to pay fees to the collection agency, which may be 30% to 40%. So the amount collected (if it is indeed collected) will be significantly reduced from the balance you are owed. Second, there is a risk that being taken to a collection agency may anger and alienate the client and result in the filing of a licensure board complaint or malpractice suit, which is perhaps related to a previously undiscussed grievance (leading to the unpaid balance) which they are now airing. While they might not prevail, especially if you have informed them in the initial agreement that unpaid bills may be sent to a collection agency, having to respond to a licensing board complaint or malpractice suit can be very costly in terms of time, stress, and expense. For these reasons we suggest taking the loss, learning the lesson of not allowing an unpaid balance to build up, and not pursuing collections actions.

WHEN A CLIENT DOES NOT WANT TO USE THEIR INSURANCE

Consider this scenario. You are a contracted Blue Cross provider. Jane Doe comes to see you for psychotherapy and she is a Blue Cross subscriber. Sounds simple enough, as you are an in-network provider that accepts her insurance. However, she tells you that she does not want to use her insurance to pay for psychotherapy and that she will pay out of pocket. She provides several reasons for making this decision. First, her employer reviews all medical expenditures for the company each year. She does not want to risk her employer finding out that she is seeking psychotherapy and has a diagnosable mental disorder (e.g., Major Depression). Second, she does not want her husband to know she is talking with a counselor, as she is contemplating divorcing him, and he is occasionally violent. The Explanation of Benefits form from Blue Cross is mailed to her residence and there is a chance her husband will open this piece of mail. She does not want to risk his becoming upset. Third, at some point in the future she wants to apply for life insurance and she does not want there to be a paper trail anywhere that indicates that she had been involved in mental health counseling, as she believes (rightly or wrongly) that having a history of a diagnosable mental condition and having had treatment for it might render her uninsurable.

For whatever reason, there are times when a client will not want to use the health insurance they have paid for to offset the costs of mental health services. So what is a mental health professional to do in such a situation? Say to Ms. Doe, "Sorry, but I cannot see you because I am required to take your Blue Cross insurance?" It is essential to understand the contract that you have signed with the carrier. Some may preclude seeing Ms. Doe and insist that you refer her to another clinician who is not a Blue Cross provider. Others may not say anything about this and the clinician may see Ms. Doe, respecting her decision not to use her insurance. If the contract is unclear, we suggest that the clinician clarify in writing with the insurer (without providing the client's name) that there is no reason that you cannot see that client.

In such cases we would also recommend that the clinician have Ms. Doe sign a brief statement that reads something like this:

I understand that I have health insurance that includes mental health benefits through Blue Cross. However, I am choosing not to use my insurance to help pay for the costs of counseling and that I authorize Dr. Public to bill me directly for services at his usual and customary rate. I confirm that I will not attempt to become reimbursed by Blue Cross at a later date. In the future I may decide to change this arrangement and choose to use my insurance to help pay for subsequent counseling sessions. If so, I will inform Dr. Public in writing, and I will be responsible for costs that are not covered by my carrier such as applicable deductibles and copays.

_____

Signature   Date

The purpose of such a document is twofold. First, it acknowledges that the client is voluntarily choosing to bypass using their insurance coverage and work directly with Dr. Public at his usual rate. This precludes anyone from later indicating that the clinician used undue influence to have the client pay for services at a higher fee-for-service rate, rather than their discounted insurance rate. Second, at times clients may indicate they do not want to use their insurance but later change their mind. They would then ask the clinician for a Superbill documenting dates of service, diagnosis, service provided, and fee charged. If this were submitted later, the insurer might (a) decline payment because services were not authorized or they were submitted past the contracted filing period (often 60 days), or (b) pay for the services but at the contracted rate because the clinician was an in-network provider. The clinician would then be expected to provide a refund to the client for the difference between the contracted rate and the rate they were paid by the client, which was probably not a discounted rate. If payment for services is declined due to a late filing, then the clinician would owe back monies previously paid by the client, because by contract clinicians cannot bill for unauthorized services.

As can be seen in the preceding statement, clients may later change their minds and decide to use their insurance to help pay for services. This request should be done in writing and be honored by the clinician.

MEDICARE

For most insurance carriers a clinician can decide to become an in-network provider and then make application to be a participating provider. If they do not want to be a provider for that MCO, they do not have to do anything. However, Medicare regulations present a different scenario. If you want to be a provider for Medicare, you complete the application and await approval. You may then start seeing Medicare patients and bill for services accordingly. However, if you do not want to participate in Medicare, but still want to see these beneficiaries, a clinician has to proactively "opt out" of being a Medicare provider. Clinicians may not legally see Medicare patients fee for service if they have not opted out. Further, those who have previously participated in Medicare who no longer wish to do so may withdraw from participation as an in-network provider.

Harris (n.d.) addresses the issue of a Medicare subscriber wanting to pay for services out of pocket, rather than using their benefits. If the clinician is a Medicare provider, according to Harris, they are precluded from accepting these patients on a fee-for-service basis. That is, they must use their Medicare benefits to pay for services, and the regular contracted fee schedule must be in place. Medicare contracts with several fiscal intermediaries who administer the program locally and may have varying administrative policies. The opt-out documents must be submitted to these groups.

INFORMING CLIENTS ABOUT THE NATURE AND LIMITATIONS OF THEIR INSURANCE

Clients are frequently misinformed about their insurance benefits. All they typically know is that they may have a deductible to meet each year and have a copay that may be due for each office visit. To further compound their confusion, mental health benefits may be different from their other health care benefits. There may be separate deductibles, coinsurance that is due at a different percentage, and even a separate company that their insurance has carved out to administer the benefits. For example, large companies or insurers may carve out or subcontract all of their mental health benefits to MCOs such as Magellan or Value Options. All a client typically knows is that on the front of their insurance card it indicates they have a Blue Cross plan, and may not be aware that on the back of the card it indicates a separate number for behavioral health or substance abuse benefits.

As part of fully informed consent it is the ethical responsibility of mental health clinicians to discuss insurance issues with each client. This is part of informing clients as early as feasible in the treatment relationship regarding their financial commitment to seeking out services. This also includes informing the client on the initial telephone call if you do or don't participate in their insurance plan so they do not arrive for a visit with false expectations. Many times your name may be on a provider list years after you have discontinued your participation with a particular carrier.

Clients must provide written permission for the clinician to bill their insurance carrier for services. Clients should also be encouraged to discuss their benefits, and specifically any limitations to their benefits, with their insurer as early as possible. Despite the passing of parity laws, there are still exceptions or special circumstances that result in differential treatment of mental versus physical health benefits by some insurance plans. For example, there is no limit on the number of sessions that a client may have in visiting a physician. However, there may be limits on their mental health benefits. Clients rarely have to obtain preauthorization to see a physician. However, some insurers require that preauthorization be obtained to see a mental health professional. Further, they reserve the right to review treatment records and retrospectively ask for a refund if they believe medical necessity has not been reached. In these cases, the clinician cannot then ask the client for reimbursement, as by contract they may not be reimbursed for services that are not deemed medically necessary.

For those psychologists who provide psychological testing services where insurance is involved, preauthorization may be required before the carrier reimburses these services. The MCO may or may not pay for parts of the process that the psychologist deems necessary for a competent evaluation. For example, they likely will not pay for time spent in (a) review of records, (b) interviewing relevant collaterals (e.g., teachers, parents, psychotherapists), (c) going to a meeting with a physician or school Individualized Education Program team to explain the results, or (d) preparing an extensive report.

For these reasons, it is imperative that psychologists be intimately familiar with the contract they sign with the MCO, have open communication with it, and openly discuss the limitations (if any) that the MCO will place on the evaluation process. Psychologists should carefully review and understand the contract to include how the MCO defines medical necessity and their policy for delivering services and charging for these services if they are determined to not meet their criteria for medical necessity. For example, if the MCO only authorizes 4 hours to complete an evaluation, but the psychologist takes 8 hours to do so, they typically will not be reimbursed for the additional hours spent. On the other hand, some MCOs allow the psychologist to provide such services and bill the client directly at the contracted rate for the services. In such cases it is essential that the psychologist (a) receive confirmation that they may do so from the MCO in each case, or else risk an accusation of being out of compliance with their contract; and (b) have the client sign a statement that they understand that the services being provided have been determined by their MCO to be medically unnecessary, but that they still want the psychologist to provide the services and that they will pay the psychologist for them.

What is essential for clinicians to keep in mind that it is they themselves, and not the MCO, are responsible for delivering a service to the client. The MCO has responsibility for providing access and payment for what it deems medically necessary. Clinicians have the responsibility for competent delivery of services. As such, if the MCO places restrictions on the way a psychologist completes the evaluation, we suggest that the psychologist think long and hard about whether or not to complete the evaluation.

For example, if the psychologist believes that administering an MMPI-2 is essential to answer the referral question, then they must administer an MMPI-2. If the MCO says that you cannot do so, or that reimbursement for such testing will not be forthcoming from either the MCO or the client, the psychologist should either (a) administer the MMPI-2 on a pro bono basis or (b) decline the referral. In short, the psychologist must still do a competent job regardless of payment for completing the work. At times psychologists are called upon by a licensing board, ethics committee, or malpractice attorney to be accountable for their involvement in a case that "went wrong." They would not want to be in the position of being asked the question, "Well, Dr. Public, you thought this client should be administered an MMPI-2, but you chose not to do so. Can you explain why not?" An answer of, "Well the MCO wouldn't pay me for it" is likely to result in an adverse outcome for the psychologist. It is better to decline an evaluation request than to do it incompletely due to a financial decision by an MCO.

For those psychologists who provide psychological testing services where insurance is not being used, it is important to explain to clients all of the costs that will be incurred in completing an evaluation. The clinician may charge for testing, scoring the tests, completing a clinical interview, interviewing collaterals, reviewing relevant records, writing a report, and having a feedback session in which the findings are communicated and discussed. If the client does not have insurance it is essential that the psychologist inform the client at the beginning of the evaluation the approximate total costs. Some psychologists charge a flat fee for such an evaluation, whereas others charge an hourly fee. If the latter method is used the client should not be surprised or have "sticker shock" when the evaluation is completed and they are presented with a bill. Psychological reports may be a few pages or they may be extremely long, depending on the nature of the referral question being answered in the evaluation, the context in which it is being written (e.g., forensic vs. a consultation to a primary care physician), and the preferred writing style of the psychologist. It may take the psychologist 1 hour to write or dictate a report, or it may take them up to 10 to 12 hours. If the psychologist charges their usual hourly fee for writing a report that takes 10 hours, the evaluation may be quite costly. This does not mean the psychologist cannot ethically charge for their time, but rather that the client needs full disclosure from the beginning.

ACCURATE BILLING

Walfish and Barnett's (2009) 15th Principle of Private Practice Success states, "Although not to the point of having a disorder, it is helpful to have some obsessive-compulsive tendencies when dealing with insurance companies and collecting payments from clients" (p. 126). There are practical reasons for focusing on billing accurately. Billing and collecting is a tedious task that takes focus and follow-through. Although inaccurate (as well as untimely) billing can impact the financial health of a clinician's practice, there are many ethical and legal issues that emerge for clinicians that may place their license, their practice, and in some extreme cases their ability to "live free and prosper" at risk.

It is an instructive exercise to do an Internet search on the terms *psychologist* and *insurance fraud*. Numerous links emerge in such a search. One would think that given all that it took to obtain a doctorate, become licensed, and develop a private practice, that no one would ever risk all of this by committing insurance fraud. Unfortunately, this is not the case. Lest we not pick on psychologists, a search on the terms *insurance fraud* and *social workers, marriage and family therapists,* and *counselors* also yields numerous links. Table 5.1 presents some of the stories that we found during our search on these terms. Fraud happens, and as you can tell from these vignettes, the penalties are steep.

Barnett and Walfish (2011) suggest that financial pressures, especially for those participating on insurance panels, may tempt the private practitioner to bill for services that have not actually been provided. There may also be a temptation to misrepresent the services that are provided, or the actual clinical diagnosis of the client, in order to obtain reimbursement at all or at a higher level. Keefe and Hall (1999) found that some practitioners believe it is necessary to report treatment needs in ways that will assure reimbursement or authorization, rather than in ways that accurately describe the client's actual clinical presentation. Insurance companies may not provide coverage for the full range of mental health services, or payment for all of the services that are provided to a client in the context of the professional relationship.

For example, as part of the informed consent process clinicians may inform clients that they may be charged for a late cancelation or a failure to show up for a scheduled appointment. This charge should be billed to the client directly and not to the insurer. Submitting a claim for individual psychotherapy to a carrier for a session that did not actually take place would be fraudulent. Clients should also be made aware of, and agree to, the amount they are to pay in these situations as part of the informed consent process.

Table 5.1 Accounts of Insurance Fraud by Mental Health Practitioners From an Internet Search

---

"Missouri Psychologist Sentenced for $1M Health Care Fraud"
"[She] was sentenced by U.S. District Judge Howard F. Sachs to three years in federal prison without parole. The court also ordered [her] to pay $1 million in restitution to Medicaid and Medicare. [She] was a licensed psychologist and private practitioner who provided psychotherapy services to recipients of both Medicare and Medicaid in their homes in the Lebanon area. On August 16, 2012, [she] pleaded guilty to health care fraud and to forgery."
http://www.insurancefraud.org/IFNS-detail.htm?key=15572#.UddYrG3krkc

"Social Worker [in] Toms River Sentenced to Prison for Health Insurance Fraud"
"A licensed clinical social worker was sentenced to 90 days in the Ocean County Jail and five years of probation for fraudulently billing insurance companies for services she did not perform.... In pleading guilty on Sept. 12, [she] admitted that between Jan 3, 2003 and Nov. 22, 2008, she fraudulently obtained money from Horizon Blue Cross Blue Shield of New Jersey and Guardian Life Insurance Co. by submitting claims for professional services she did not provide. The investigation began after one of [her] former clients received an Explanation of Benefits document from his health care insurance company indicating that [she] had submitted claims for payment for more than twenty counseling sessions that had not taken place."
http://www.newjerseynewsroom.com/healthquest/social-worker-mary-rizzuto-of-toms-river-sentenced-to -prison-for-health-insurance-fraud

"Former South Jersey Therapist Sentenced to Prison for Submitting Fraudulent Bills for Services to Insurance Company"
"A former South Jersey family and marriage therapist was sentenced to state prison today for engaging in fraudulent billing by submitting approximately $22,000 in bills to an insurance company for services that he did not provide.... [His] license was suspended by the New Jersey Board of Marriage and Family Therapy Examiners.... In pleading guilty, [he] admitted that between Aug. 20, 2004 and March 21, 2006, he fraudulently submitted more than $22,473 in bills to Cigna Behavioral Health Insurance Company for therapy services."
http://www.nj.gov/oag/newsreleases12/pr20120601b.html

"[North Carolina] Counselor Found Guilty of Medicare Fraud"
"[She] was accused of participating in a scheme for two years to submit claims for Medicare counseling services that never were performed.... Prosecutors alleged that [she], a licensed professional counselor who was approved by Medicare to provide mental and behavioral health services, conspired with [two other clinicians], who were not licensed, to submit claims under [her] name and provider number.... A number of Medicaid recipients testified during the weeklong trial, which ended Friday, that they or their children never received the therapy services that [she] claimed to have pro-vided.... Evidence submitted during the trial also showed that [she] routinely billed for more than 24 hours of therapy services in a single day. For one day in December 2009, the government claimed, [she] submitted claims for 69 hours of services.... [She] faces up to 35 years in prison and a fine of up to $750,000.
http://www.insurancefraud.org/IFNS-detail.htm?key=15693#.Uddemm3krkc

Many insurance companies will not pay for couples' psychotherapy, which is CPT Code 90847. When clients or clinicians want to "get around" providing this noncovered service, they may inappropriately bill the insurance carrier for individual psychotherapy (CPT Code 90834) instead, as this is a covered service. There may be pressure from the couple who financially feel the need to have their insurance pay for the service and who may not be able to pay privately. The couple would then either not have counseling, or have to go to a lower-fee social service agency for these services. The psychotherapist may not feel like they are doing anything wrong because they have a couple in front of them that is in distress and in need of help and the insurer would pay for individual psychotherapy anyway. However, to do so would be fraudulent.

In their survey of practicing mental health professionals, Pope, Tabachnick, and Keith-Spiegel (1987) found over one third of their sample viewed altering a diagnosis in order to receive reimbursement by an insurance carrier as unethical. However, over one fourth of the sample acknowledged having done so in the past, with over one third doing so on a frequent basis. For example, many clients go into psychotherapy for personal growth reasons. That is, they do not have an actual disorder that merits a diagnosis. However, insurance carriers will likely not pay for personal growth psychotherapy, as they only provide coverage for diagnosable disorders that meet the standard of medical necessity. Although it may seem relatively innocuous to assign a diagnosis of Adjustment Disorder, NOS, it (1) would be fraudulent to do so and (2) ignores the fact that there is no such thing as an innocuous mental health diagnosis, as this may have later implications for the client for obtaining certain types of insurances, security clearance, or jobs. As another example, many insurers will not pay for a V-code diagnosis such as Parent-Child Communication Problem. Because of this, to receive reimbursement from an insurer, the clinician may assign the child a diagnosis of Oppositional Defiant Disorder (because they are a behavior problem) or Depression (because there "must be" an underlying depression to account for the misbehavior). However, to do so would be fraudulent and what Barnett and Walfish (2011) and Gresham (2009) have discussed as client–psychotherapist collusion against the insurance company.

Psychologists often employ psychometrists to conduct psychological testing for them under their supervision. The CPT Code for Psychological Testing with Report (by a Psychologist) is 96101, and the CPT Code for Psychological Testing by a Technician is 96102. The reimbursement rate for the former code is often much higher than for the latter code. Because of this, psychologists at times have submitted billing forms to insurers in which it appears they have done the testing, when in fact the testing was conducted by their psychometrist. When consulting with us about billing issues, one psychologist recently stated, "Well, how can I make any money when they reimburse so little for psychometrists?" Although sympathetic to the situation, we informed this colleague that this was fraudulent practice (the psychologist was unaware of this and indicated that "everyone in town does it this way") and he decided to no longer offer this service in his practice. It was not financially viable and he certainly did not want to consciously do something that was ethically and legally incorrect.

In a similar vein, mental health professionals often take on associates in their practice as they expand from a solo to a group practice. If a clinician's practice has been successful they may have overflow or a waiting list that they can refer to their associates. Although associates can be sources of revenue for the practice owners—and in our experience this is a typical motivator for expanding one's practice—oftentimes associates, especially when they come into the practice, may not be on any (or all) of the insurance panels on which the practice owners participate as a contracted provider. There may be a temptation for the professional who is a provider for the insurance carrier to submit a claim with their name on the form, implying that they provided the services when in fact their associate did so. As has been highlighted, this is an unethical behavior and likely constitutes insurance fraud.

Additionally, at times associates, especially early career professionals, may not be licensed to practice independently. Indeed, they may have joined the practice with the goal of gaining supervised work experience that would count as practice hours necessary to be able to become licensed. Note that one of the fraud examples presented in Table 5.1 was of a licensed mental health professional who had unlicensed clinicians provide care. The licensed professional submitted claims to the insurer as if it were they who provided the service, rather than the unlicensed clinician. When a claim is submitted to the insurance carrier with a clinician's name as the providing professional, there is an attestation that it is the professional that personally provided the service and not a supervisee or another clinician. As such, submitting a claim on behalf of a clinician who is not licensed, to include a supervisee accumulating hours for licensure, is likely to be considered inaccurate representation of billing and therefore unethical, as well as illegal fraudulent behavior.

Note that there are some exceptions to the preceding behavior being fraudulent. First, there are some insurers who in some cases will allow reimbursement for supervised practice. However, before assuming that this will be allowed, we recommend that the supervising clinician contact the insurer or MCO in writing (not by telephone because a paper trail should be established in case of later accused misinterpretations) and specifically ask them this question. Their answer should be received in writing and no services related to this question delivered prior to it being received. Second, if you are a "group practice" you may bill under one tax ID number. However, each member of the group has to be credentialed by the insurance carrier and is still making the same attestation that they personally provided the professional service rendered. It is highly unlikely that many will credential someone who is not licensed, but this is something to be confirmed in writing with each carrier. Third, one may be able to bill for supervised services if the practice becomes or actually is "a clinic." That would require a different corporate structure and applying to the local jurisdiction (or possibly county) to become a mental health clinic. In these instances just the clinic is credentialed and not individual clinicians. The owners of the clinic would be responsible for the care that is provided, but we speculate that all of the clinicians do not have to be licensed. Of course there are requirements to become a licensed mental health clinic; an application has to be completed, and then reporting requirements that may be in place for authorized clinics complied with. Becoming a clinic is accompanied by added administrative costs and administration time to ensure compliance with regulations and that quality services are being provided.

Last, as part of accurate billing and collecting, there are times when overpayments are made to clinicians by clients for services provided. This may occur if a client did not think they met their annual deductible or a client miscalculates their copay due. In these instances clinicians are obligated to refund the monies due in a timely manner to the client who made the overpayment. At times these overpayments are made by insurance carriers. Some clinicians might be tempted not to mention it to the insurance carrier, hoping they never realize the mistake. They would only return the monies if requested. Other clinicians might credit the client's account, because these monies were paid on behalf of the client by the carrier. We have known other clinicians to actually send the check to the client, assuming these are their monies and any refund due is between them and the insurance company. All of these can lead to problems later, as the refund should go back to the insurer as the entity that made the overpayment. The point is we should not keep money that is an overpayment and instead should return it to the source, whether it is the client or the third-party payor.

NOT ALL INACCURATE BILLING IS DUE TO FRAUD OR DECEIT

Barnett and Walfish (2011) acknowledge that at times inaccurate billing occurs as a result of the mental health professional wanting to take the easy way to get rich or to scam the system. However, billing errors may occur as a result of the busy mental health professional (a) being careless, (b) having insufficient oversight over employees, or (c) lacking knowledge of how to bill appropriately.

We once completed a psychological evaluation and thought we had billed for 4 hours of CPT Code 96101 (Psychological Testing With Report). However, when we received a check from the insurer for more than $4,000, we knew that a mistake had been made somewhere. The billing program was checked, and it was learned that 41 units of testing had been billed rather than 4! Rather than quickly cashing the check and heading off for vacation, we returned the check to the insurer with an explanation and a request to process a corrected claim. Please note that insurance companies are not likely to become upset if you have found a mistake in billing and quickly rectify it. It can be understood that mistakes happen. However, they do not understand, or have little tolerance for, mistakes not being corrected quickly.

Most people conceptualize fraud as billing for a service that has not been provided. However, insurers also retain the right to audit charts of the clinician who has contracted to be a provider for them (though the extent of this audit may be restricted by law in some states, and this will be discussed later) to determine if appropriate documentation has been provided to justify the medical necessity of the service being provided. It is essential that clinicians become familiar with the documentation required by each insurer with which they have signed a contract. In addition, they should become familiar with the audit procedures outlined in the contract. It is also important that documentation be completed in a timely manner, as it may be difficult to know how much time you spent with a client in session one week later.

The federal government makes a special effort to recoup medical expenditures that they believe have been paid due to waste and fraud. Harris (n.d.) cites data from a government report indicating that in reviews of Medicare beneficiaries' treatment records, "47% of the claims did not meet Medicare requirements, 26% of the claims were miscoded, and 19% were insufficiently documented" (p. 3). A colleague recently reported that he had been audited by the Recovery Audit Program, a group that conducts audits of Medicare claims to identify overpayments to providers. He described that he had a small part-time practice, primarily serving Medicare patients. The audit resulted in a judgment of a refund of $5,000 to the government as a result of inadequate documentation. He described, "Well, my charting wasn't the best, and I didn't want to get into a long and drawn-out fight, so I just wrote the check." So although he did provide the service, he was still asked to refund the monies paid to Medicare because he had not adequately documented that the services provided were medically necessary. At a minimum one's record keeping should reflect the symptoms and history indicating the need for services. These then should tie to the specific diagnosis and criteria needed for making the diagnosis. A statement of the rationale and plan for assessment and treatment should be clearly documented. It is important to be aware that clinical records may be examined at a later time; thus, when documenting, mental health professionals should keep in mind the goals and the potential uses of their documentation. In essence, there is a strong tie and compatibility among good clinical practice, good ethical practice, and good business practice.

It is the responsibility of the clinician to provide adequate oversight of their employees. Most mental health professionals do not do their own billing and collecting. Rather, they delegate this process to staff, a family member, or a billing service with which they contract. Barnett and Walfish (2011) describe the pros and cons of contracting with a billing service. The key ingredients in making this decision rest in the value placed on time by the clinician, the degree of need for direct control of the process, level of tolerance for others' mistakes, and willingness to take on a tedious and laborious task. However, if the billing and collection process is delegated, the clinician is still legally and ethically responsible for the task and the behavior/performance of those performing the task on his or her behalf. In addition to knowing these parties are qualified to do the task, practitioners are also responsible for ongoing supervision and review to ensure that the tasks support staff completes continue to be provided in a competent and ethical manner (Barnett, Cornish, Goodyear, & Lichtenberg, 2007). Such staff (paid or volunteer) should also sign a HIPAA Business Associate Contract that specifies their obligations to protecting each client's confidential information. See the website of the U.S. Department of Health & Human Services at (http://www.hhs.gov/

ocr/privacy/hipaa/understanding/coveredentities/contractprov.html) for Sample Business Associate Contract Provisions.

It is easy to have a lack of knowledge of how to bill appropriately that results in an ethical or legal transgression. No one that we know of took a class is graduate school titled, "Billing 101." However, because they are billing and collecting for services provided, private practitioners are obliged to be aware of the procedural steps, as well as the ethical issues, involved in appropriate billing and collecting.

Billing and collecting can be a complicated process when the clinician is being paid by an outside third party. As we said earlier, it is essential that you carefully review and understand the contracts that you sign with each MCO. This review should take place before you sign the contract. Other parties for which you or your staff members provide services such as workers compensation, vocational rehabilitation services, or employee assistance programs may have their own idiosyncratic rules and regulations. For example, one colleague reported that billing and reimbursement methods for workers compensation clients are different in two states in which he has practiced. The rules from one state did not generalize to the other state. Thus, each mental health professional must become educated on the rules for submitting claims in their local jurisdiction with each individual company with which they have a contract.

Rules about CPT codes must be followed carefully. In our consulting work we have learned about a clinician who routinely went over his 1-hour sessions by 15 minutes, so after four sessions he billed for another hour session. His logic was that he provided an hour's worth of service, so therefore he was entitled to bill for this time. Unfortunately, this faulty logic led to the loss of his license to practice because he billed for sessions that did not occur (he had to make up a fictitious date in order to bill for the 60 minutes). All services provided should be billed accurately, regardless of the reasoning used for considering the use of "creative" billing strategies.

INFORMATION TO BE COMMUNICATED TO MANAGED CARE ORGANIZATIONS

Broskowski (1991) has argued that MCOs developed as an outgrowth of concern regarding costs and quality of care provided in the mental health industry. Clinicians clearly do not like managed care interfering with their practice or income (e.g., Cohen, Maracek, & Gillham, 2007; Keefe & Hall, 1998; Phelps, Eisman, & Kohout, 1998), and Walfish and O'Donnell (2008) found in a survey of clinicians that relationships with MCOs were rated as being the most stressful aspect of being in private practice.

As we have noted, it is essential that each clinician be aware of what is asked of them in their MCO contracts. Certain documentation is required on each client. Psychotherapy session notes may need to include certain information. Billing information needs to include date of service and an accurate diagnosis. Requests for authorization of psychological testing may require a working diagnosis, reasons why the testing is being requested, and a description of relevant history. With this information the MCO can decide if it is going to authorize payment for testing. There are some MCOs that will authorize an initial set of sessions (e.g., 6–10) but then require that the clinician complete a form to request continuing treatment or conduct a peer review over the telephone.

As part of the informed consent process, clinicians must also educate their clients regarding the type of information the MCO can request about themselves. Clients also need to provide written consent to the clinician prior to this information being shared with the MCO. Clients need to understand that payment for services may depend upon the release of this information. Some clients may not want to have this information shared and may choose either not to use their insurance to pay for services (see related section hereafter) or not enter into treatment in the first place. If the insurer asks a question that you believe the client might object to you answering (e.g., the insurer wants detail about a sexual trauma), you can always postpone answering the question until you have had time to consult with the client. The client and you may risk not getting reimbursed, but you also might avert the possibility of avoiding a breach in the relationship with the client due to a lack of informed consent about the disclosure.

If psychotherapists feel uncomfortable sharing detailed clinical information with the MCO, or feel it is unethical to do so, we suggest that consideration be given as to whether or not to participate in managed care. Walfish and Barnett's (2009) 18th Principle of Private Practice Success urges clinicians who participate in managed care to accept it with all of its limitations and ramifications, exactly as it is and not how they think it should be, in order to reduce frustration and dissatisfaction. Reinforcement for this principle is found in a study by Acker and Lawrence (2009), who found social workers who felt competent to practice in a MCO environment experienced lower levels of role stress and burnout.

It is important to note that the information MCOs request from clinicians is being tested in the courts at the time of this writing in a suit filed by the New Jersey Psychological Association. Information about the suit may be found at https://www.psychologynj.org/advocacy/legal-action-initiative and Axelbank (2012). As Axelbank describes the basis for the suit, psychologists in New Jersey believe that the information the MCOs are requesting violates both the State Licensing Law by requiring clinicians to violate patient confidentiality, and the New Jersey Peer Review Law, which limits the type of information (limited to demographics, dates of service, diagnosis, setting in which the services are provided, voluntary–involuntary status, reason for continuing treatment, and prognosis), that may be released to third parties about patients.

DENIAL OF CARE BY AN INSURER

If a clinician requests additional sessions to work with a client because they believe there is a medical necessity to justify continued treatment, and the MCO denies payment for the sessions, what is a practitioner to do? They see a clinical necessity, yet there may be no funds to pay for treatment. As noted, Younggren and Gottlieb (2008) do not believe that psychotherapists should have to work for free. In discussing this issue Barnett (1993) states that clinicians "must be sensitive to their responsibility to avoid premature termination of treatment, despite the denial of authorization to provide further care" (p. 161). Barnett (1993) summarizes literature to suggest that the onus of demonstrating that abandonment did not occur with a particular client may fall on the psychotherapist.

Once again it is essential to be aware of the details of the contract that you sign with the MCO. Newman and Bricklin (1991) point to the need for the psychotherapist to appeal a denial of authorization of payment for services, if such a decision is contrary to the clinical judgment of the clinician. Turchik, Karpenko, Hammers, and McNamara (2007) review significant court decisions and conclude that clinicians cannot simply acquiesce to the decision of the MCO, and must appeal the denial. If this appeal is denied, the details of the contract should outline options available to meet the client's treatment needs. If the MCO has deemed further treatment to not be medically necessary, such rules may (a) preclude the contracted clinician from seeing the client at all because mental health services have not been found to be medically necessary; (b) include a clause that allows the clinician to see the client at the contracted rate, but the client will be responsible for the entire fee; or (c) include a clause that allows the clinician to see the client at whatever rate the client and contracted clinician agree upon. Cooper and Gottlieb (2000) point to the need for the clinician to be aware of the rules of the MCO and have a plan in place for their client should authorization of payment be denied. This may mean seeing the client pro bono until stabilized (if not contractually prohibited) or making a referral to a social service agency or training clinic where the client may be seen on a sliding scale or low-fee basis. Barnett (1998) simply states that "utilization reviewers may only refuse to authorize payment for additional treatment. They may not deny you the right to provide treatment. If a patient is in crisis, treatment must be provided" (p. 21). Thus, regardless of MCO authorizations, clinicians must fulfill their responsibilities to their clients when continued treatment is clinically indicated, either by providing that treatment themselves, or through appropriate referrals.

One of the authors has had success in appealing a denial on a complicated case with a patient who had multiple suicide attempts but was being denied weekly visits, as the patient was then more stable. When speaking directly with the person doing the review, the clinician stated that the conversation with the reviewer was being documented, as was the clinician's statement to the reviewer that the lack of payment would probably lead to the patient terminating treatment, becoming more symptomatic and actively suicidal. He went on to say that should the appeal not be overturned this statement would certainly be in the record and available should there be legal action in the future. The appeal was successful. The mere verbalization of the procedure of documentation and its probable impact seemed to be the deciding factor, as no new clinical information was provided on the appeal.

ETHICAL CHALLENGES

- Clients need full disclosure about financial issues in order to make an autonomous decision about entering into treatment, yet many times clinicians are hesitant to discuss these matters.
- Taking into consideration a client's ability to pay for the services that are needed may present challenges in treatment planning.
- Efforts to develop a strategy for providing a sliding scale fee arrangement may prove challenging when a third-party payor deems it inappropriate to do so.
- Raising fees is one of the few ways clinicians have to earn more money in private practice. However, it must be done in a way that allows sufficient notice for clients to make informed decisions, is not financially exploitive, and does not ignore a client's clinical needs.
- There are many insurance carriers with different types of programs within each company. It is important to be familiar with the details of each contract that you sign and its implications for the financial relationship you have with your client.
- Clinicians are allowed to utilize collection agencies for unpaid bills, but must do so following regulatory and ethical standards.
- Consistent accurate billing is difficult to achieve but important to strive for. Inaccurate billing may lead to ethical or legal transgressions.
- Managed care organizations request information to determine medical necessity of treatment, but at the same time it is important to preserve client confidentiality.
- Although an insurance carrier may deny payment for services, the mental health professional must attend to the clinical needs of the client.

KEY POINTS TO KEEP IN MIND

- Resolve the possible conflict of altruism and being a small business owner.
- Inform clients as early as possible about fees and payment policies.
- Not all clients can afford to pay full fee for services.
- The buildup of a large balance due is likely as much a clinical and administrative issue, as it is an issue of a client not being responsible.
- When a client makes an autonomous decision not to use their insurance to pay for services, it is important to know the details of your contract with the insurance carrier.
- The government is making a concerted effort to recover funds from clinicians for services deemed medically unnecessary.
- Documentation of services provided, especially with Medicare clients, needs to be done consistently with prevailing standards for detail and accuracy.

- Contractual language with an insurer may be difficult to understand because these contracts are written by attorneys. These contracts are written in the best interests of the insurance carrier and not the clinician who may sign the contract. It is important to read these contracts carefully and even have them reviewed by an attorney if needed to make sure you understand what you are being asked to sign. It is far too late to read the contract after it is signed.
- Learning how to do accurate billing is a detail-oriented task, and although it may be delegated, the responsibility still lies with the clinician for ensuring that it is done accurately and consistently within ethical standards and legal requirements.
- Every insurance carrier has different criteria and procedures for documenting medical necessity of services.
- Awareness of ethical and legal requirements for amount and type of client information that may be shared with insurance carriers is essential.

PRACTICAL RECOMMENDATIONS

- Have an easy-to-read and comprehensive Informed Consent for Treatment agreement, and provide a sufficient focus on informed consent issues related to fees, billing, and payment expectations.
- Anticipate that some clients may experience financial difficulties during the course of treatment that impact their ability to pay for services. Address this possibility and how it may be addressed in the informed consent process.
- For business and humanitarian reasons, consider reserving some psychotherapy hours for low-fee or pro bono clients.
- Place information about possible increases in fees in the initial Informed Consent to Treatment documents and then discuss with clients when this will occur, providing them with adequate notice should it provide a hardship for them and create the need to make alternative arrangements.
- Collect payments due at the time that services are provided to prevent the buildup of a large balance due.
- Develop a form that clients sign when they choose not to use their insurance to pay for services.
- Find out from each insurance carrier what documentation is needed to demonstrate medical necessity of services and what type of correspondence is required.
- Learn how to do billing, even if you delegate the task to someone else, providing sufficient oversight when these tasks are delegated.
- Maintain a list of necessary criteria for determining medical necessity of services for each insurance carrier, as well as appeal procedures if services are denied.

PITFALLS TO AVOID

- Thinking that informed consent can simply be relegated to providing a client with a written document for them to sign.
- Assuming that because a client says they can afford your services, that they actually can afford your services.
- Tailoring the client's course of treatment and modality of treatment solely to their ability to pay. Treatment planning and decisions should be guided primarily by the clinical needs of the client.
- When trying to be altruistic, sidestepping contractual obligations or the law.
- Placing personal financial goals ahead of a client's clinical needs.
- Being reluctant to talk to clients about monies that are due for services rendered.
- Assuming that your preferred mode of documentation of services provided meets the standards of the insurance carrier that you have contracted with.
- Signing a contract with the intention of following your own clinical and procedural preferences, when they may be inconsistent with what is allowed by the contract.
- Failing to appeal adverse utilization review decisions when your clinical assessment indicates the need for ongoing treatment for the client.

RELEVANT ETHICS CODE STANDARDS

Fees and Informed Consent

- AAMFT Code of Ethics (AAMFT, 2012) Principle 7, Financial Arrangements, states, "Marriage and family therapists make financial arrangements with clients, third-party payors, and supervisees that are reasonably understandable and conform to accepted professional practices" (p. 4).
- ACA Code of Ethics (ACA, 2005) Standard A.10.b, Establishing Fees, states, "In establishing fees for professional counseling services, counselors consider the financial status of clients and locality" (p. 6).
- APA Ethics Code (APA, 2010) Standard 6.04a, Fees and Financial Arrangements, states that as "early as is feasible in a professional or scientific relationship, psychologists and recipients of psychological services reach an agreement specifying compensation and billing arrangements" (p. 9). Additionally, Standard 6.04b states, "Psychologists' fee practices are consistent with law," and Standard 6.04c states, "Psychologists do not misrepresent their fees" (p. 9).
- NASW Code of Ethics (NASW, 2008) Standard 1.13(a), Informed Consent, states, "When setting fees, social workers should ensure that the fees

are fair, reasonable, and commensurate with the services performed. Consideration should be given to client's ability to pay" (p. 9).

Collections

- AAMFT Code of Ethics (AAMFT, 2012) Principle 7.3, Financial Arrangements, states, "Marriage and family therapists give reasonable notice to clients with unpaid balances of their intent to seek collection by agency or legal recourse" (p. 4).
- ACA Code of Ethics (ACA, 2005) Standard A.10.c., Nonpayment of Fees, states, "If counselors intend to use collection agencies or take legal measures to collect fees from clients who do not pay for services as agreed upon, they first inform clients of intended actions and offer clients the opportunity to make payment" (p. 6).
- APA Ethics Code (APA, 2010) Standard 6.04(e), Fees and Financial Arrangements, states, "If psychologists intend to use collection agencies or legal measures to collect unpaid fees, psychologists must first inform the person that such measures will be taken and provide that person an opportunity to make prompt payment" (p. 9).
- NASW Code of Ethics (NASW, 2008) Standard 1.16c, Termination of Services, states, "Social workers in fee-for-service settings may terminate services to clients who are not paying an overdue balance if the financial contractual arrangements have been made clear to the client, if the client does not pose an imminent danger to self or others, and if the clinical and other consequences of the current nonpayment have been addressed and discussed with the client" (pp. 4–5).

Accurate Billing

- AAMFT Code of Ethics (AAMFT, 2012) Principle 7.4, Truthful Representation of Services, states, "Marriage and family therapists represent facts truthfully to clients, third-party payors, and supervisees regarding services rendered" (p. 4).
- ACA Code of Ethics (ACA, 2005) Standard C.6.b, Reports to Third Parties, states, "Counselors are accurate, honest, and objective in reporting their professional activities and judgments to appropriate third parties including, courts, health insurance companies, those who are recipients of evaluation reports, and others" (p. 10).
- APA Ethics Code (APA, 2010) Standard 6.06, Accuracy in Reports to Payors and Funding Sources, states, "In their reports to payors for services . . . psychologists take reasonable steps to ensure the accurate reporting of the nature of the service provided . . . the fees, charges, or

payments, and where applicable, the identity of the provider, the findings, and the diagnosis" (p. 9).

- NASW Code of Ethics (NASW, 2008) Standard 4.04, Dishonesty, Fraud, and Deception, states, "Social workers should not participate in, condone, or be associated with dishonesty, fraud, or deception" (p. 16). Further, NASW Standard 3.05, Billing, states, "Social workers should establish and maintain billing practices that accurately reflect the nature and extent of services provided and that identify who provided the service in the practice setting" (p. 14).

Terminating Treatment When There Is a Lack of Insurance Authorization

- AAMFT Code of Ethics (AAMFT, 2012) Principle 1.11, Non-Abandonment, states, "Marriage and family therapists do not abandon or neglect clients in treatment without making reasonable arrangements for the continuation of treatment" (p. 3).
- ACA Code of Ethics (ACA, 2005) Standard A.11.a, Abandonment Prohibited, states, "Counselors do not abandon or neglect clients in counseling" (p. 6). Further, Standard A.11.d., Appropriate Transfer of Services, states, "When counselors transfer or refer clients to other practitioners, they ensure that appropriate clinical and administrative processes are completed and open communication is maintained with both clients and practitioners" (p. 6).
- APA Ethics Code (APA, 2010) Standard 10.10c, Terminating Therapy, states, "Except where precluded by the actions of clients/patients or third-party payors, prior to termination psychologists provide pretermination counseling and suggest alternative service providers as appropriate" (p. 13).
- NASW Code of Ethics (NASW, 2008) Standard 1.16b, Termination of Services, states, "Social workers should take reasonable steps to avoid abandoning clients who are still in need of Services" (p. 10).

REFERENCES

Acker, G., & Lawrence, D. (2009). Social work and managed care: Measuring competence, burnout, and role stress of workers providing mental health services in a managed care era. *Journal of Social Work, 9,* 269–283.

American Association for Marriage and Family Therapy. (2001). *Code of ethics.* Retrieved from http://www.aamft.org/imis15/content/legal_ethics/code_of_ethics.aspx

American Counseling Association. (2005). *ACA code of ethics.* Retrieved from http://www.counseling.org/Resources/aca-code-of-ethics.pdf

American Psychological Association. (2010). *Ethical principles of psychologists and code of conduct.* Retrieved from http://www.apa.org/ethics

Axelbank, J. (2012). Smoke in our offices: What can we do? *Independent Practitioner, 32*, 42–44.

Barnett, J. E. (1993). Ethical practice in a managed care environment. *The Independent Practitioner, 13*, 160–162.

Barnett, J. E. (1998). Termination without trepidation. *Psychotherapy Bulletin, 33*, 20–22.

Barnett, J. E., Cornish, J. E., Goodyear, R. K., & Lichtenberg, J. W. (2007). Commentaries on the ethical and effective practice of clinical supervision. *Professional Psychology: Research and Practice, 38*, 268–275.

Barnett, J. E., & Johnson, W. B. (2008). *Ethics desk reference for psychologists.* Washington, DC. American Psychological Association.

Barnett, J. E., & Walfish, S. (2011). *Billing and collecting for your mental health practice: Effective strategies and ethical practice.* Washington, DC: APA Books.

Bennett, B. E., Bricklin, P. M., Harris, E., Knapp, S., VandeCreek, L., & Younggren, J. N. (2006). *Assessing and managing risk in psychological practice: An individualized approach.* Rockville, MD: The Trust.

Broskowski, A. (1991). Current mental health environments: Why managed care is necessary. *Professional Psychology: Research and Practice, 22*, 6–14.

Cohen, J., Maracek, J., & Gillham, J. (2007). Is three a crowd? Clients, clinicians, and managed care. *American Journal of Orthopsychiatry, 76*, 251–259.

Cooper, C. C., & Gottlieb, M. C. (2000). Ethical issues with managed care: Challenges facing counseling psychologists. *The Counseling Psychologist, 28*, 179–236.

Gresham, M. (2009). Ethics and fees in practice. *The Independent Practitioner, 29*, 100–101.

Harris, E. (n.d.). Issues with reimbursement under Medicare. Retrieved from http://www.apait.org/apait/resources/articles/medicare.pdf

Keefe, R., & Hall, M. (1998). Managed care's impact on the financial well-being of social workers in private practice. *Social Work in Health Care, 28*, 11–29.

Keefe, R., & Hall, M. (1999). Private practitioners' documentation of outpatient psychiatric treatment: Questioning managed care. *Journal of Behavioral Science Research, 26*, 151–170.

Martin-Causey, T. (2005). Building your dream practice from the ground up. In J. E. Barnett & M. Gallardo (Eds.), *Handbook for success in independent practice.* (pp. 59–65). Phoenix, AZ: Psychologists in Independent Practice.

National Association of Social Workers. (2008). *Code of ethics.* Retrieved from http://www.socialworkers.org/pubs/code/code.asp

Newman, R., & Bricklin, P. M. (1991). Parameters of managed mental health care: Legal, ethical and professional guidelines. *Professional Psychology: Research and Practice, 22*, 26–35.

Phelps, R., Eisman, E., & Kohout, J. (1998) Psychological practice and managed care: Results of the CAPP practitioner survey. *Professional Psychology: Research and Practice, 29*, 31–36.

Pope, K. S., Tabachnick, B. G., & Keith-Spiegel, P. (1987). Ethics of practice: The beliefs and behaviors of psychologists as therapists. *American Psychologist, 42*, 993–1006.

Turchik, J. A., Karpenko, V., Hammers, D., & McNamara, R. (2007). Practical and ethical assessment issues in rural, impoverished, and managed care settings. *Professional Psychology: Research and Practice, 38*(2), 158–168.

Walfish, S., & Barnett, J. E. (2009). *Financial success in mental health practice: Essential tools and strategies for practitioners.* Washington, DC: APA Books.

Walfish, S., & O'Donnell, P. (2008). Satisfaction and stresses in private practice. *The Independent Practitioner, 28,* 135–138.

Woody, R. H. (1988). *Fifty ways to avoid malpractice: A guidebook for mental health professionals.* Sarasota, FL: Professional Resource Exchange.

Younggren, J. N., & Gottlieb, M. C. (2008). Termination and abandonment: History, risk, and risk management. *Professional Psychology: Research and Practice, 39,* 498–504.

6

Staff Training and Office Policies

Hiring staff, whether licensed professionals or administrative, presents unique ethical challenges. These individuals represent you and your practice and extend your exposure and liability as they interact on your behalf, both in and outside the workplace. The training, vigilance and ongoing staff development initiatives that you provide can go a long way toward creating a practice that routinely performs in an ethically sensitive manner.

GENERAL PROFESSIONALISM

Setting a tone of professionalism can help create a culture that is careful to avoid ethical pitfalls. Behavioral health practices can be stressful environments for all staff. In some practices there can be tendencies to tell stories, joke, and even make fun of certain clients. This may be done from the standpoint of "easing the tension" rather than being mean spirited. However, a lack of professionalism can, in our opinion, heighten the practice's ethical exposure. If the practice owners routinely behave in a professional manner, staff members learn that the culture is one that does not tolerate unprofessional behavior. Many inadvertent ethical "slips," such as discussing a patient in earshot of other patients, can be avoided by staff viewing themselves and their roles in a professional way and recognizing that inadvertent ethical slips can be damaging to the patient, a third party (e.g., someone overhearing a conversation about someone else), and the practice.

CONFIDENTIALITY, CONFIDENTIALITY, CONFIDENTIALITY

It is often said, "The three most important things in real estate are location, location, location." In a behavioral health practice, when it comes to staff and ethics, the three most important things are *confidentiality, confidentiality, confidentiality.* Although there can be other ethical violations, it often seems that confidentiality slips are the easiest to make and are at times based on subtle disclosures or inadvertent mistakes.

It is easy to make mistakes. Sometimes there can be social pressure to disclose information (e.g., when a major referral partner starts discussing a case in common with you, but you do not have a release). At other times, you may feel more of an internal urge to disclose information (such as thanking a referral partner without first getting a signed release). In all cases, it is much better to exercise care to avoid such behaviors.

Confidentiality is also breached inadvertently in many other ways. It is important to be vigilant and teach clinical and administrative staff to take great care and avoid the following frequent errors:

- Using patient names when discussing a patient on the telephone, in the waiting room, in the hall, or in public.
- Keeping last names in written or electronic calendars.
- Taking records out of the office.
- Leaving files or billing information face up on a desk.
- Assuming that because your office door is closed no one can hear you.

In general, a good approach is to teach all staff to protect patient identity and related clinical information as they would their own wallet. Would they leave their wallet on their desk when they step away for a few minutes? Would they leave a purse open in front of others? Would they read their credit card number aloud while others in the waiting room might be able to overhear the number? Teaching staff to think about the patient's identity as truly *protected* information (U.S. Department of Health and Human Services, 1996) can help avoid unintentional disclosures.

DELEGATION TO SUBORDINATES

Typically, when we think of "delegation," we think that we are moving the responsibility for something to someone else. Similarly, we often feel or assume the responsibility for a task when it is delegated to us. However, in the context of professional practice, delegation does not lessen responsibility. It actually multiplies the responsibility by the number of people who have responsibility through the chain of command. Moreover, it also increases the risk as more people are now involved in a situation, each of whom can cause an error.

For example, let's look at a practice where there is one clinician who has 50 open cases at any time over the course of a year. If that clinician makes one accidental error when it comes to the security of records over the course of the year (e.g., leaving a file cabinet unlocked), the practice has an exposure of that one error per year. If that same clinician owns a group practice with six associates and three administrative staff people, and we assume each of the staff might make one error per year, that same clinician (now owner of the practice) has ultimate responsibility for 10 errors per year. The chance of an actual breach of confidentiality is now more likely, as the same file cabinet (or file room) might now be left unlocked 10 times per year instead of once. As the business owner, you remain responsible. Your ultimate responsibility for ethical violations has implications for what you choose to delegate, as well as for how you ensure competence, and how you supervise professional and administrative staff.

Consequently, delegation to subordinates needs to be done with great care and attention to detail. For example, create procedures such as an end-of-the-business-day office lockup checklist (see end of chapter for a representative example), which can be implemented routinely so behavioral habits develop that reduce the likelihood of ethical violations. Then, be vigilant and check to make sure those procedures are being followed regularly. Offer staff constructive feedback when there are problems or the practice is exposed to a potential compromise in ethics. These situations become learning opportunities for the staff member who is involved, as well as for other staff. Attention to office and record security also can be a behavior that is evaluated in the staff member's annual performance review.

Delegation to subordinates also has another ethical wrinkle: It is easy to put subordinates in a situation that it is outside their skill set. The owner of a practice may have great zeal to get work done, secure a practice opportunity, and help less seasoned professionals try new things. Likewise, staff members (clinical or administrative) want to please the practice owner. This can cause excessive demands for performance, rushing, and a loss of situational awareness, which again can lead to inadvertent ethical compromises (e.g., inappropriately sending out confidential information, or calling a patient by name in front of other patients, etc.).

BOUNDARIES AND RELATIONSHIPS

Issues around boundaries and relationships can be complex, subtle, and varied. It also can be difficult to predict the ability of staff to discern the risks related to the management of boundaries and relationships. This can be especially problematic for administrative staff, who are likely to have less awareness and training about these issues and who see themselves as just being friendly as they strike up casual conversations with clients in the waiting room. Unfortunately, they may not readily recognize that this casual conversation can be psychologically evocative or embarrassing for the patient or family member and be experienced as a boundary violation.

Administrative staff members should not be expected to innately and clearly understand the subtleties of boundaries and relationship issues. After all, they have not completed graduate-level training in a mental health field and have not taken courses in ethics. It is the responsibility of the mental health professional to provide ongoing education regarding these issues. There is a fine line between staff members being friendly and courteous to clients in the waiting room (which is essential in developing an atmosphere where clients want to come for treatment), and crossing boundaries or becoming friends or romantically involved with clients or their family members. For example, we have been involved in a situation in which a staff member and client shared an enthusiasm for a certain college football team. These discussions led to the staff member and the client attending a game together. Mental health professionals understand this is clearly inappropriate behavior. However, administrative staff may not understand the issues involved, and therefore it must be made explicit that administrative staff and clients may not socialize with each other. In rural communities this is a particular challenge, as the focus often needs to be on how staff will behave when they unavoidably encounter clients outside of the office.

Also, don't assume that your professional staff members have the same ethics training and sensitivities as you do. Your practice is not theirs and their risk tolerance may not at all be the same as yours.

Professional and administrative staff members need to be encouraged to bring questions regarding boundaries and relationships to supervisors, and there need to be multiple discussions to sort out the most appropriate actions. Practice owners and supervisors can model sensitivity to, and open discussion of, these issues by bringing similar concerns that they have to clinical and administrative staff meetings for discussion and input.

It is also important to consider one's relationships with staff and especially subordinates when thinking about boundaries and relationships. The authors have heard many complaints from both early-career mental health professionals and administrative staff about inappropriate humor, sexualized innuendo, and touching from supervisors and practice owners as well as from the professional staff toward the administrative staff. Such behavior is inappropriate and can cause grave individual and systemic problems in the workplace. It may also be illegal, leading to grievances, fines, and lawsuits, which are unlikely to be covered by malpractice insurance and to which individuals who are found guilty may be at substantial personal financial risk. Our ethics do not just apply to our interactions and dealings with patients; they also apply to our behavior with colleagues and staff.

SECURITY OF RECORDS AND THE FACILITY

Provisions need to be made for the safe storage of records and for the facility itself to be safe. We have previously discussed the need to safeguard records in the office setting and to secure electronic equipment with passwords. Staff members should not take client records or billing information home in the evening or over the weekend. Office doors can have locks installed and not be left open when staff is out to lunch or away from their desks. Backups of files can be made and safely secured. Here again, relevant policies and practices can be in place to assure for safety of records. All professional and administrative staff members need to be trained to follow your security measures on a routine basis and comply with HIPAA policies and requirements.

Security also applies to emergency situations. In private practices such events can be very rare; however, it is important to prepare for these as well. If you practice in an office building suite and the fire alarm rings, what are the procedures for protecting clients and personnel as well as computers and patient records? These procedures should be written down and in place in advance of a problem. Similarly, procedures should be in place if there is a clinical emergency in the suite. Establishing a procedure, including it in personnel policies, and reviewing it periodically (e.g., annually) can go a long way toward protecting clients and the records of their treatment (Fisher, 2009).

For example, if the fire alarm is sounded, there can be a simple routine of locking file cabinets and shutting off computers (without waiting for programs to close, even if it means losing some of the day's data) and exiting the suite and building (making sure patients are escorted out as well). A common meeting place can be assigned in advance (perhaps across the street from the building) so that an attempt can be made to account for all people who were in the suite.

The fire alarm may sound far more frequently than simply when there is a fire (e.g., when the building owners are testing the system, or if there is a false alarm). Of course, one needs to treat each alarm seriously and react accordingly. However, if only some people leave the office suite, and if records are left out and computers left on, any people who remain in the suite (such as a person who refused to leave during what seemed like a drill) or arrive at the suite (such as emergency personnel) will have complete access to the confidential information, which could have been protected by taking just a few seconds to turn a switch or push in a file cabinet lock.

In a clinical emergency, such as a threatening patient in the waiting room, a suicidal patient on the phone, or a potentially violent patient in the office, a code word or phrase known to all staff can be used to indicate that there is an emergency situation that will require a call to 911. Some practices will make up a name of a doctor who is not affiliated with the practice and have a phrase such as, "Can you please tell Doctor [name] that his wife called?" This lets the other staff know that there is an emergency that requires outside help, without necessarily alerting others and causing a panic or escalation of the problem.

As with other situations, the key in emergencies is to prepare in advance to reduce the risk of injuries and mishaps. Clear and well-thought-out procedures that are documented and periodically reviewed can help make sure that ethical concerns are addressed even on these relatively rare occasions.

POLICIES AND PROCEDURES: A SAFETY NET

"We're a family here." "I hire good people." "We all trust each other." "We're experts at having difficult conversations." These are some sample comments from practice owners as they describe their practice and the rationale for not having written policies and procedures. However, most corporate employment law attorneys will tell you that written policies and procedures are a cornerstone to protecting a business (i.e., your practice) when it comes to complaints. Written policies and procedures can demonstrate that you are concerned about the possibility of an ethical breach and have taken steps in advance to educate all employees about the potential and how you want them to respond. Written policies also become a reference for employees when there may be some confusion. They can be teaching tools for orienting new employees.

The employee's responsibility to follow the practice's policies and procedures can be described in an employment agreement or letter of hire as a condition of employment. This can further set the expectation that you take this seriously and that you want to make sure there is an explicit understanding of this expectation at the time of hire. Clearly this is as important as specifying the number of vacation days, compensation, and other features of the job.

If there is a violation or breach of ethics and you determine that you want to begin some type of internal remediation, these clauses in your agreement can be part of the basis and justification for insisting on a course of action if the employee wants to maintain employment. Of course, as with other important practice matters, the complaint, evidence obtained, and actions taken should be in writing so that there is a documented history of your actions. You can even have a policy outlined in a policy manual that describes a procedure that includes due process and progressive discipline for handling a complaint.

Consider a scenario where a senior clinician is acting inappropriately with a student or staff member. There is no written policy that is tied to an employment agreement and you have not documented what actions you have taken when this was brought to your attention. However, you have handled the situation and believe it resolved. Some time later there is a second incident with the same senior clinician. The employee who is impacted goes to an outside agency and files a formal grievance or complaint. You have no information specifying your policies and how you have "handled" the situation. It can easily be construed that nothing was done and that you thereby condoned the inappropriate behavior—and now a "pattern" of such behavior—by the senior staff person. Now, consider the same scenario but add in the written policy tied to the employment agreement and documentation around your investigation and actions in response to both complaints. There may still be a negative outcome for the practice, but you will likely be in a much better situation and be able to show that you took steps to address the problem and were not negligent. Your business and employment records can be as important as your clinical records.

In short, staff development is an ongoing process of training and education to foster continued attention to the business, clinical, and ethical obligations and challenges inherent in providing mental health services.

ETHICAL CHALLENGES

- Staff discussing a patient in earshot of the waiting room or other patients.
- Releasing information about a spouse without adequate formal releases.

- Confidential documents left where others may view them.
- Staff discussing cases with other staff, family, etc.
- Mailing, faxing, or e-mailing one client's information to another in error.
- Quickly responding to a request from a lawyer because it looks official, serious, and complete on first glance.
- Assuming professional and administrative staff have the same ethical sensitivities as you.
- Assuming interest demonstrated by staff equates to clinical or administrative competence.
- There are many situations that have complex and subtle factors, which may put others in situations where their risk of being (or feeling) exploited increases.
- It is difficult to train staff to an appropriate response for every potential boundary or relationship problem that may occur.
- Staff may not readily recognize a boundary problem or seek input when a potential problem presents itself.
- Consistently following all security procedures is difficult to ensure. One error is all it takes for a breach to occur.
- Staff needs to be trained in routine and emergency procedures.

KEY POINTS TO KEEP IN MIND

- Don't allow staff members to work in a bubble. Professional and administrative staff members need to be trained to seek multiple sources of input around ethical challenges and dilemmas. Such discussions can help raise consciousness and awareness of risk factors, sort out options on a particular situation, and create a practice culture where seeking input is the norm. Input is often the key to effective risk management around ethically challenging situations.
- Written policies and procedures are important to have in place so that staff is informed and the risk of inadvertent ethical violations is reduced.
- One of the best ways to avoid an ethical breach is to get input. Staff needs to be encouraged to seek input whenever they have doubt about a situation.

PRACTICAL RECOMMENDATIONS

- Develop a culture that reinforces professionalism.
- Train staff members on their first day of work about professionalism, confidentiality, boundary issues, security and emergency procedures, and the policies you have related to these issues.
- Train all staff in how to call a patient's home or work without compromising confidentiality.

- Train administrative staff how to appropriately ask for payment, address patients, and pursue accounts receivables.
- Train professional staff how to address informed consent for treatment and a discussion of office policies and confidentiality during their first clinical visit.
- Encourage frequent discussions about ethical concerns and a nonpunitive open-door policy for professional and administrative staff to ask questions and raise *any* ethical concerns, dilemmas, and problems.
- Consider developing a brief quiz to ensure that staff members understand policies and procedures as they relate to confidentiality, record security, and relationships with clients and boundaries (see end of chapter for a sample quiz).
- Stay vigilant and address relatively small or potential transgressions.
- Continue to educate staff about ethical situations that arise and appropriate courses of action.
- Immediately and directly address an ethical problem when it arises.
- Establish written policies for calling patients by name, maintaining document security, having private conversations with doors open, using sound screens, keeping names in calendars, and the like. Tie these policies to written employment agreements for all professional and administrative staff. Make sure staff members sign a statement indicating they have received these policies and will follow them as a basic requirement of their position. Review your polices and procedures and update them as needed on an annual basis.
- Freely offer apologies when a violation has occurred and actively take steps to correct the problem(s).
- Develop routine procedures and standards of practice. Monitor compliance in self and others.
- Bring issues that you face to administrative and clinical staff meetings so as to encourage discussion and model the behavior you are looking for in others.
- Make sure your clinical staff members follow through with having clients sign an informed consent form, which mentions the limits to security (e.g., emails, and voice mails).
- Develop emergency procedures to protect patients, staff, and the confidentiality of records.

PITFALLS TO AVOID

- Jokes, stories, and nonprofessional behavior in general.
- The absence of a written employee agreement for all employees and staff that specifies they need to follow all of the practice's written policies and procedures as a condition of employment.
- The absence of written policies and procedures that highlight the expectations for employees regarding key ethical behaviors.

- Leaving an open appointment book on the desk in the waiting room.
- Discussing confidential information in front of other clients.
- Leaving charts to be filed later out on the desk or counter where clients may access them.
- Not spending time adequately training staff and assuming they have the necessary training in ethically sound decision making based on their prior experience.
- Staff members may develop personal relationships over time with patients/ clients. This can even apply to administrative staff who may get to know people who come to the office on a regular basis.
- Assuming mistakes won't happen.
- Assuming professional staff will know the proper course to take to avoid ethical problems.
- Denying or covering up mistakes that have occurred.
- Assuming low-likelihood events (e.g., your car won't be broken into when there are records inside or a patient left alone in the waiting room won't peek at a computer that is on) won't occur.
- Falsely representing the security of emails, voice mails and other systems where confidential information may reside.
- Assuming that issues around boundaries and relationships do not apply to colleagues and staff members.

RELEVANT ETHICS CODE STANDARDS

Delegation to Subordinates

- AAMFT Code of Ethics (AAMFT, 2012) Principle 4.4, Oversight of Supervisee Competence, states, "Marriage and family therapists do not permit students or supervisees to perform or to hold themselves out as competent to perform professional services beyond their training, level of experience, and competence" (p. 5).
- ACA Code of Ethics (ACA, 2005) Standard B.3.a., Subordinates, states, "Counselors make every effort to ensure that privacy and confidentiality of clients are maintained by subordinates, including employees, supervisees, students, clerical assistants, and volunteers" (p. 7).
- APA Code of Ethics (APA, 2010) Standard 2.05, Delegation of Work to Others, states, "Psychologists who delegate work... take reasonable steps to (1) avoid delegating such work to persons who have a multiple relationship with those being served that would likely lead to exploitation or loss of objectivity; (2) authorize only those responsibilities that such persons can be expected to perform competently on the basis of their education, training or experience, either independently or with the level of supervision being provided; and (3) see that such persons perform these services competently" (p. 5).

- NASW Code of Ethics (NASW, 2008) Standard 3.03, Performance Evaluation, states, "Social workers who have responsibility for evaluating the performance of others should fulfill such responsibility in a fair and considerate manner and on the basis of clearly stated criteria" (p. 6).

Boundaries and Staff Relations

- AAMFT Code of Ethics (AAMFT, 2012) Principle 3.8., Harassment, states, "Marriage and family therapists do not engage in sexual or other forms of harassment of clients, students, trainees, supervisees, employees, colleagues, or research subjects" (p. 4). Further, Principle 3.9, Exploitation, states, "Marriage and family therapists do not engage in the exploitation of clients, students, trainees, supervisees, employees, colleagues, or research subjects" (p. 4).
- ACA Code of Ethics (ACA, 2005) Standard C.6.a., Sexual Harassment, states, "Counselors do not engage in or condone sexual harassment. Sexual harassment is defined as sexual solicitation, physical advances, or verbal or nonverbal conduct that is sexual in nature, that occurs in connection with professional activities or roles, and that either 1. is unwelcome, is offensive, or creates a hostile workplace or learning environment, and counselors know or are told this; or 2. is sufficiently severe or intense to be perceived as harassment to a reasonable person in the context in which the behavior occurred. Sexual harassment can consist of a single intense or severe act or multiple persistent or pervasive acts" (p. 10).
- APA Ethics Code (APA, 2010) Standard 3.03, Other Harassment, states, "Psychologists do not knowingly engage in behavior that is harassing or demeaning to persons with whom they interact in their work based on factors such as those persons' age, gender, gender identity, race, ethnicity, culture, national origin, religion, sexual orientation, disability, language or socioeconomic status" (p. 6). Further, Standard 3.02, Sexual Harassment, states, "Psychologists do not engage in sexual harassment" (p. 6).
- NASW Code of Ethics (NASW, 2008) Standard 2.01a, Respect, states, "Social workers should treat colleagues with respect" (p. 5). Further, Standard 2.07a, Sexual Relationships, states, "Social workers who function as supervisors...should not engage in sexual activities or contact with...colleagues over whom they exercise professional authority" (p. 5).

Security of Records

- AAMFT Code of Ethics (AAMFT, 2012) Principle 2.4, Protection of Records, states, "Marriage and family therapists store, safeguard, and dispose of client records in ways that maintain confidentiality and in accord with applicable laws and professional standards" (p. 3).

- ACA Code of Ethics (ACA, 2005) Standard D.1.e., Establishing Professional and Ethical Obligations, requires counselors who work with others to "clarify professional and ethical obligations of the team as a whole and of its individual members" (p. 11).
- APA Ethics Code (APA, 2010) Standard 4.01, Maintaining Confidentiality, states, "Psychologists have a primary obligation and take reasonable precautions to protect confidential information obtained through or stored in any medium" (p. 7).
- NASW Code of Ethics (NASW, 2008) Standard 1.07l, Privacy and Confidentiality, states, "Social workers should protect the confidentiality of clients' written and electronic records and other sensitive information. Social workers should take reasonable steps to ensure that clients' records are stored in a secure location and that clients' records are not available to others who are not authorized to have access" (p. 3).

REFERENCES

American Association for Marriage and Family Therapy. (2012). *Code of ethics*. Retrieved from http://www.aamft.org/imis15/content/legal_ethics/code_of_ethics.aspx

American Counseling Association. (2005). *ACA code of ethics*. Retrieved from http://www.counseling.org/Resources/aca-code-of-ethics.pdf

American Psychological Association. (2010). *Ethical principles of psychologists and code of conduct*. Retrieved from http://www.apa.org/ethics

Fisher, M. A. (2009). Ethics based training for nonclinical staff in mental health settings. *Professional Psychology: Research and Practice, 40*, 459–466.

National Association of Social Workers. (2008). *Code of ethics*. Retrieved from http://www.socialworkers.org/pubs/code/code.asp

U.S. Department of Health and Human Services. (1996). Health Insurance Portability and Accountability Act of 1996. Retrieved from http://www.hhs.gov/ocr/privacy/

ETHICS QUIZ FOR STAFF

Please answer the following items "True" or "False."

1. When a patient's wife calls to confirm her husband's appointment time, it is okay to give her the information. [False: You do not know if the wife even knows the patient is in treatment or if there is a release on file. You also do not know if the person calling is indeed the patient's wife.]
2. When a mother calls to confirm whether her teenage son attended his session this afternoon, it is okay to give her the information. [False: The teenage son's presence in treatment may be confidential and you may not know if the mother has a legal right to the information.]
3. It is better practice to not leave a message that this is "Dr._____ calling...." [True: Leaving such a message might expose the patient's presence in treatment to a family member or those in the workplace.]
4. When sending a letter to a patient's home, it is better to have a return address that does not directly identify the sender. [True: Having a nondescript return address can protect the patient's presence in treatment.]
5. If professional staff is discussing patients in earshot of the waiting room it is okay, because the professionals know what is best. [False: They may not know what is best and may not even realize they are putting themselves, the practice, and the patient they are discussing at risk.]
6. It is okay to leave paperwork with client information on your desk or computer screen for just a few minutes if you have to step away. [False: It only takes a minute for there to be a violation of confidentiality. It is best to at least temporarily put the information out of sight.]
7. You should not use a patient's last name when calling on the phone if you are in earshot of others. [True: Others may hear the call and the content and know who the patient is, thereby breaching confidentiality.]
8. You should not use a patient's last name when calling on the phone until you are certain you have actually reached the patient. [True: You may have dialed wrong and could be releasing information about the patient's presence in treatment.]
9. You should rip up billing or other information and put it in a closed plastic garbage bag when disposing of it. [False: Although ripping up the information is better than not doing so, the information should be shredded.]

10. Ethical situations have clear answers and if you don't know the answer, you should ask a colleague. [False: Asking for input is good, but you should ask the owner(s) of the practice, as ultimately it is their decision about the appropriateness of the action given the clinical situation and the way they want to run the practice.]

END-OF-THE-BUSINESS-DAY LOCKUP CHECKLIST

☐ Do not leave the office if any patient files or any other materials that might identify a client (e.g., telephone messages not yet in a file) are left unsecured in any part of the office. Be sure all patient files are put in file cabinets and that the file cabinets are locked with the keys put away in a secure location.

☐ Place any appointment scheduling books in a secure location such as in a locked file cabinet. Do not leave them laying out where others may be able to access them.

☐ Be sure all computers are logged off and all programs are shut down. Do not just trust the presence of a screensaver to ensure the security of private materials on computers.

☐ Check photocopiers, fax machines, wastepaper baskets, and the like for any papers or other materials with patient information on them. Be sure all such materials are shredded prior to leaving the office.

☐ Ensure that all doors are locked (e.g., file room, treatment rooms, main door to the office) as you leave for the day.

7

Advertising and Marketing

As business owners and operators, in order to promote our venture successfully and to ensure that new practice opportunities are generated on an ongoing basis, private practitioners must engage in advertising and marketing activities. Failure to do so will likely result in an unsuccessful enterprise. Mental health professionals should implement effective business strategies to promote their practices in an ethical and appropriate manner. Good ethics are good for business just as excellence in clinical skills is good for business. A balance must be struck between promoting our work and ensuring that our prospective clients are not taken advantage of or harmed in any way. As such, it is important that each practitioner is knowledgeable about the ethics standards relevant to the advertising and marketing of our practices, and that we implement them in accordance with these standards.

ADVERTISING AND PUBLIC STATEMENTS

How we represent ourselves to the public and to our referral partners is of great importance. It is vital that prospective clients know of us, the services we provide, our credentials and training, and any other information that may be of relevance to them when seeking out professional services. At a minimum, we will want to ensure that information about us and our practices is both accurate and readily available to the public. This can include the traditional "yellow pages" ad or advertisements in other publications such as newspapers and magazines, your business card and letterhead, the use of a website and blog to advertise and promote your practice, and the use of online referral networks or services, among others. Regardless of the medium used, there is some basic information that must be shared with the public, but sharing it accurately and ethically is key.

At a minimum it is important to share your name, highest relevant academic degree, professional title and/or licensure status, the range of services you provide, special training or expertise and certifications you may have, information on fees and participation in insurance networks, location and possibly directions, and accessibility for the disabled. It is essential that information shared with the public be accurate, up to date, relevant, and objectively presented.

Sharing Credentials

To the general public, the more initials and letters after a professional's name, the more skilled or better trained they will perceive the professional to be. Of course, in reality this is not necessarily the case. Mental health professionals should only list their highest earned degree that is relevant to the professional services being provided. For example, if a professional has a PhD in theology from a past career but has a MS in counseling psychology and is advertising as a counseling professional, it would be a misrepresentation to the public to list "MS, PhD" after their name. Only the MS degree should be listed, as someone may assume that the PhD is in the counseling field. In this example the doctorate in theology is not relevant to the provision of mental health services or to one's status as a licensed counselor.

In addition to sharing licensure status and professional certifications earned, mental health professionals should be cautious about listing "vanity board" certifications. The accepted standard is only to list those board certifications that involve an evaluation of the professional's clinical competence and expertise. Certifications that in essence simply require the payment of a fee to receive a certificate and certification can be seen as a misrepresentation to the public, because they will likely view this credential as indicating advanced competence in the profession (Datillo, Sadoff, & Gutheil, 2003). In the profession of psychology the most widely accepted board certification credential is provided through the American Board of Professional Psychology (ABPP). ABPP offers the board certification credential in 14 areas of psychology practice. Detailed information about the ABPP board certification process can be found at www.abpp.org.

Implying or Promising Specific Results or Outcomes

One issue related to advertising one's services to the public concerns not taking advantage of the public's trust and vulnerability. Often, individuals who are seeking mental health services are in crisis. Their ability to effectively evaluate information presented to them may be limited. Thus, mental health professionals should avoid all subjective evaluative statements about the services they provide, statements about the quality of services offered, and anticipated outcomes from participation in treatment. One would therefore not make statements such as, "Best Psychotherapy Services in Town," "Achieve the Best Results Possible Here," or "Join our Depression Busters program and start achieving happiness today!"

Even the name one selects for their mental health practice is an important aspect of the advertising of yourself and the services you provide. A practice named "Greater Baltimore Mental Health Associates" or "Atlanta Medical Psychology

Group" shares information with the public about the general geographic region served by the practice and the nature of services provided. However, practices named "Optimal Mental Health Outcomes" or "Center for Effective Counseling" have implications for the public that go beyond factual information, and thus should be avoided.

If a mental health professional possesses unique training or qualifications, these would be appropriate to announce because this would be the sharing of factual information. For example, a clinician that is certified in the use of hypnosis by the American Society of Clinical and Experimental Hypnosis may appropriately advertise as "ASCEH Certified in Clinical Hypnosis." If it is factually accurate, they could also state, "Specializing in the treatment of pain, smoking cessation, and weight loss with hypnosis." But it would be unethical and a misrepresentation to the public if in his or her advertising, this mental health professional stated, "Recognized expert in the treatment of pain, smoking cessation, and weight loss with hypnosis, the most effective treatment known."

It is also important to avoid advertising that preys on the public's fears or vulnerability. For example, the following would be an inappropriate advertisement:

Is your adolescent ever moody or withdrawn? Is he or she ever argumentative or uncooperative? Does he or she seem secretive and tend to avoid family interactions? Depression is a serious mental health concern that affects thousands of adolescents and that can ruin one's life if left untreated. But, help is available. If you fear that your adolescent may suffer from depression contact the Adolescent Treatment Center today so that your adolescent can begin receiving the help he or she needs.

Parents who are struggling to understand their adolescent, even if displaying what may be typical behaviors for that stage of development, may be so concerned that, when reading this advertisement, they may easily conclude that their child may be depressed, that depression is a very serious condition, and that their child is in need of immediate treatment. Such an advertisement goes far beyond providing factual information objectively, and would likely be seen as exploitative and inappropriate.

TESTIMONIAL ENDORSEMENTS

One form of advertising that mental health professionals may consider is the use of testimonial endorsements that are provided by current or former clients. Testimonial endorsements are used in advertising in a wide range of businesses. For example, they are frequently seen in automobile sales and service commercials in which an apparently satisfied customer tells about how wonderful their experience with that particular dealership or service center has been. We have also seen such advertising by attorneys, physicians, and chiropractors, among others. This can be a very effective form of advertising because the public may view the testimonial endorsement of a customer as more meaningful or valuable to them than statements made by the business owners themselves. The testimonial endorsement, even if provided by a complete stranger, may seem more like a recommendation or referral from a trusted friend or family member.

But the relationship between an automobile salesperson and their customer is very different from the relationship between a mental health clinician and a psychotherapy client. The nature of the professional relationship with clients is very different from all other relationships clients have in their lives. The counseling relationship is by design a one-sided relationship, with the focus being on the client's needs and best interests. Mental health professionals are obligated to act only with the client's best interests in mind and to ensure that all actions are consistent with the agreed-upon treatment goals and plan.

To ask a client for a testimonial endorsement places the client in an uncomfortable position. Many clients will be vulnerable to the clinician's influence and will not want to risk disappointing or alienating the clinician. The client may not truly have the ability to decline the request due to fears about how a refusal might affect future treatment and the treatment relationship. Will they feel the need to embellish or sensationalize in order to consciously or unconsciously please the psychotherapist? Even if the client offers to provide the testimonial endorsement, accepting this offer can be seen as violating or taking advantage of the client's trust. As has been stated, clients rely on their mental health clinician to act only in ways that are in the client's best interest.

To use a client's testimonial endorsement, even when the client offers it, has important implications for the client's privacy. Of course the client will understand that the testimonial endorsement will be made public through its use in advertising. However, clients may not fully understand the implications for them with regard to disclosing the existence of, and some details about, their personal psychotherapy. In an effort to please or be helpful to their clinician, clients may be risking unanticipated consequences in their lives. Thus, refusing to use testimonial endorsements from clients would be consistent with a focus on the clients' best interests and our responsibility to protect the client's privacy and avoid exploiting them.

Accepting a testimonial endorsement from a client should be seen as entering into an inappropriate multiple relationship. The clinician and client are then engaging in a separate business relationship (even though no funds are being exchanged for providing the endorsement) in addition to the treatment relationship. One must ask how this new relationship is relevant to the client's clinical needs and treatment plan. It most likely is not and only serves to meet the clinician's business needs by promoting their practice. It is also important to consider what happens if a client's treatment goes poorly after a testimonial endorsement is given. Can the client take back the endorsement? Would the endorsement cease to be accurate and now be a misrepresentation for the clinician to continue using it?

One can also consider the possible negative impact that testimonial endorsements in our advertising can have on the public. Prospective clients may be uncomfortable with the thought of being asked to serve in this role should they enter treatment. They might then decide to forego needed treatment because of this discomfort, something that can be seen as a disservice to that individual.

UNINVITED IN-PERSON SOLICITATIONS

In keeping with the admonishment against preying upon the public's vulnerability, mental health professionals should not engage in uninvited solicitations. Although we may advertise our professional services to the public at large, as we have described, it is not appropriate to seek out individuals who are emotionally vulnerable and directly solicit their participation in treatment. The treatment relationships mental health professionals have with their clients should be based on trust and respect, not on exploitation of emotional vulnerability (Barnett & Klimik, 2012).

An example of an uninvited solicitation would be for the mental health professional to spend time in funeral homes and, at the end of each funeral or memorial service, to approach individuals who are distraught and offer them counseling services. A clinician might accost individuals in this manner, offering them their business card and explaining that the loss of a loved one is very difficult to go through alone, and that the clinician specializes in helping people successfully navigate the grieving process. We hope this can be seen as very different from advertising grief counseling services to the public at large and having an individual decide independently to seek out the clinician for assistance.

As another example, clinicians often provide educational talks in the community. This is a way to provide information about mental health issues to the public. In addition, it is a way for the clinician to become known in the community. These public lectures should be viewed as imparting psychological information and not as a forum to directly solicit clients. If you are doing a talk about positive parenting and Mr. Smith starts complaining about little Johnny's behavior, it would be inappropriate to say to Mr. Smith during the lecture, "Well, Mr. Smith, I think you need to bring Johnny in to see me for a comprehensive evaluation." This would go beyond the scope of the psychoeducational lecture and be viewed as soliciting clients. On the other hand, if Mr. Smith approaches you after the lecture and says, "I'm having problems with my son, Johnny. Could we come in and see you?" by all means hand Mr. Smith one of your cards and tell him to call your office and make an appointment.

MARKETING PROFESSIONAL SERVICES

In addition to advertising, successful mental health professionals will actively market their practices both to the public and to potential referral partners. Marketing includes those activities that place the clinician in the public or referral partner's eye and that hopefully promote a favorable view of the practitioner. Examples of marketing to the public include writing a column on mental health issues and topics in a local newspaper or magazine, hosting a radio or television show on these issues and topics, and giving presentations in the local community such as at schools or to local organizations. It can also include sending letters, newsletters, announcements, and the like to potential referral partners. Each of these activities can be a part of an overall marketing plan for one's practice and, if done well, can boost referrals. However, one author has been told by other professionals that they will actively avoid referring cases to those clinicians who market in an aggressive or "slimy" fashion. Appropriate, ethical, and tasteful marketing, on the other hand, can be effective.

INTERACTING WITH THE MEDIA

In Chapter 4 we discussed some basic ethical issues when dealing with the media. To expand on this issue when writing or speaking about mental health topics through the media, it is important not to make statements that would supersede members of the public seeking out professional consultation for assessment, diagnosis, or treatment that might be needed. Articles should provide the public with general information about mental health topics of interest, but they should make it clear that the information provided should not take the place of an evaluation and treatment by a trained professional. When interacting with the public it is also important to provide general information and not offer advice or recommendations for a particular individual's situation due to not having conducted an assessment of their needs (McGarrah, Alvord, Martin, & Haldeman, 2009).

When asked questions about public figures, mental health professionals should exercise caution about making statements that go beyond their knowledge of the individual and the situation. One cannot ethically provide a professional opinion about, or diagnosis of, any individual that they have not actually evaluated. For example, you should avoid describing a politician as a sociopath or an actor as a narcissist if you have never evaluated the person. To do so is irresponsible, may have a deleterious effect on the public figure, and may also present the mental health clinician to the public in a poor light.

To help minimize the risk of ethical missteps when being interviewed by the media, it is suggested that the mental health clinician request information on the focus of the interview and possibly obtain the questions to be asked in advance to aid in the process of preparing for the interview. Being well prepared, sharing general information and not giving specific advice, and not going beyond established scientific information can help the clinician interact with the media in an ethical manner.

MARKETING IN THE COMMUNITY

Mental health professionals may build their practices by being visible in the local community and demonstrating their expertise to members of the public. Providing free workshops in venues such as to the Parent Teacher Association, civic and community organizations, and support programs such as Children with Hyperactivity and Attention Deficit Disorders (CHADD) is a way to become known to potential clients in the community. When doing so, however, it is important to ensure that only general information is provided, that no recommendations are given to individuals in the audience, and that the focus is educational. The presentation should not be seen as an opportunity to screen members of the public for treatment needs and then offer them your services. And, as was highlighted with presentations in the media, information should be shared in a manner that does not imply the presence of a professional relationship and that does not suggest that it may take the place of seeking professional treatment. Additionally, the earlier presented precautions about the use of testimonial endorsements should be kept in mind; although it is appropriate to leave handouts and business cards for attendees to pick up should they so choose, uninvited solicitations of business should be avoided.

When presenting clinical illustrations of material discussed, no actual client examples from your practice should be used unless the client has consented to this use of their confidential information. In such cases where they have given permission, identifying information and the clinical presentation must be sufficiently altered so that individuals who know the client would not be able to discern him or her from the information presented. This is especially important in a rural or small-town practice where multiple and overlapping roles and relationships may be unavoidable (Firestone & Barnett, 2012).

Marketing to Referral Partners

Marketing our services directly to potential referral partners is an essential part of each mental health professional's marketing plan. If referral partners are not aware of the services we offer and our clinical effectiveness, they likely will not refer clients to us. These marketing activities can include telephone calls and letters, visits to their offices, and even providing them with copies of articles we have written. If you want to provide work samples such as evaluation reports or summaries of successful treatments, it is important to ensure that no actual confidential client information is shared. Rather, creating a sample based on a fictitious individual (e.g., John Q. Public or Jane Q. Public) would be preferable.

Once referrals are made, many referral partners will expect periodic telephone calls or letters of update, to learn about how the client's treatment is progressing. This is a common request and a very reasonable one among health professionals. Yet an important ethical consideration is each client's privacy rights and expectations. Prior to releasing any confidential information, we must first obtain the client's informed consent, ensuring they understand the nature and extent of the release of information to be made and the reasons for doing so. Additionally, in our efforts to be helpful to referral partners it is important that we only share information relevant to their work with the client and not go beyond these needs. Sharing nonessential information that may be of a sensitive nature to the client would inappropriately violate their privacy rights.

Marketing Using Social Media

Social media is ubiquitous in our society today. Many individuals use social media such as Facebook, Twitter, and others as a primary means of communicating, sharing, and obtaining information. Because so many individuals are regularly using social media in this manner, they may be seen as outstanding means of marketing one's practice (see Kolmes, 2012 for a discussion of social media issues in different aspects of a clinical practice). Yet there are ethics concerns that come with the use of social media.

A primary concern is confidentiality. The privacy settings associated with these social media platforms are quite imperfect, and often it is very easy for individuals to learn about all others participating as well. Clinicians who use social media to market their practices may also find that clients will contact them via these media for other purposes. The line between professional and personal use of these media can easily become blurred. Further, clinicians will need to consider the potentially problematic implications of accepting "friend" requests from clients and how doing so may impact the professional relationship.

Another aspect to consider when using social media is that of boundaries between our personal lives and the amount of information that is easily accessible to our patients. Generally in a psychotherapy practice, one is very thoughtful about how and when to share personal information with a patient. For example, a male therapist may not choose to share that his wife just had a child when working with a couple struggling with infertility. Yet if this information is on a public Facebook page or the clinician announces it through Twitter or another service, the patients can easily be exposed to this information outside the session. This is not something clinicians previously had to consider. However, the importance of being thoughtful and careful about the potential negative impact of these social media disclosures should not be overlooked simply because the disclosure is happening outside the office. It is recommended that practitioners carefully consider developing a social media policy (See drkkolmes.com/for-clinicians/social-media-policy/ for an excellent example) prior to venturing into the use of social media for marketing purposes or for any other potential use with clients.

ETHICAL CHALLENGES

- Promoting your practice while not exploiting the public. Advertising and marketing activities are essential for developing and maintaining a successful mental health practice. However, we must avoid the temptation to overstate the facts, to misrepresent our credentials or services offered, or to take advantage of their vulnerability. A balance must be struck between generating business and protecting the public's welfare.

- Avoiding the temptation to use ethically questionable advertising practices. Although the use of testimonial endorsements and engaging in uninvited solicitations of business from the public may be successful in generating additional business in the short run, we must keep in mind the potential impact on the individuals involved and on the public in general. These short-term gains in business generated may come at the expense of these individual clients' welfare and the trust of the public at large. This would negatively impact the long-term success of a practice.

- Interacting with the media ethically and competently. Interactions with the media can be an important way to share our expertise with the public and can be seen as an important public service, in addition to developing one's public reputation for competence and professional expertise. But, media interactions can be tricky and one should develop competence in media interactions before embarking on these activities.

- Maintaining responsibility for all advertising and public statements made on your behalf. It is important to take the time to ensure that all statements made by you and on your behalf are accurate. When tasks are delegated it is easy for mistakes to be made. Assuming that all advertisements, promotional materials, websites, business cards, and the like will be created accurately can result in inaccurate information being shared with the public, with you responsible for these actions and their effects.

- Ensuring that all public statements and advertisements remain accurate. It is certainly appropriate to discontinue professional memberships, to not renew credentials, and the like, but it may be challenging to remember all the places where these are shared with the public. Despite these challenges, it is important to ensure that representations to the public are updated regularly as is needed to ensure their accuracy.

KEY POINTS TO KEEP IN MIND

- Although advertising is intended to generate business for your practice, it is also intended to provide the public with needed information so they can make informed decisions about what services to seek and from whom they may obtain them.

- Always represent your education, training, experience, credentials, degrees, licensure status, competencies, skills, and professional association memberships accurately.

- Never state or imply specialized expertise that has not been developed through formal education, training, and relevant professional experience.

- It is your responsibility to ensure that others are not deceived and that they understand information provided. When possible, all misunderstandings that are evident should be clarified in a timely manner.
- Present advertising material accurately and objectively, never preying on the public's vulnerability, trust, and dependence.
- Never use advertising techniques that are exploitive or take advantage of clients; testimonial endorsements should only be used with past clients and of them, only with those who are not vulnerable to your influence.
- Never promise specific results or treatment outcomes, either directly or by implication.
- When interacting with the media, ensure that information shared is accurate and based on current research and professional practice standards; refrain from commenting on particular individuals who you have not evaluated or assessed.
- When giving advice in a public forum, it should be based on accepted professional standards and only general advice should be provided. Ensure that the recipient understands that no professional relationship exists and that the general information provided should not take the place of seeking needed professional services. Such a statement should even appear on your web page.

PRACTICAL RECOMMENDATIONS

- When giving presentations, bring business cards and fliers but do not actively solicit clients.
- Do not solicit or accept testimonials from clients.
- Create a social media policy before using social media for marketing activities and carefully consider potential threats to privacy before using them.
- Double-check all marketing and publicity materials for accuracy and to avoid exaggeration or unfounded claims.
- Prepare carefully for media interviews. You can certainly ask the interviewer for the questions or scope of the interview in advance, research and plan your answers, and then contact the interviewer in a timely manner.
- Unless it is very clear from the context, ensure that all advertisements are labeled as such.

PITFALLS TO AVOID

- Sharing information with the public that is deceptive, fraudulent, or inaccurate.
- Becoming caught up in promoting your business so much that you lose sight of your responsibilities to the public by overstating or misrepresenting yourself.

- Failing to be aware of your relevant licensing law and going beyond what is legally allowed in how your represent yourself to the public.
- Failing to monitor advertisements and representations to the public over time to ensure their ongoing accuracy.
- Using advertising techniques that may be appropriate for use in other businesses but that are inconsistent with the roles and responsibilities of mental health professionals.
- Delegating responsibility for website content, promotional materials, and other advertising content to others who may not fully understand or share your focus on ethical conduct as articulated in your profession's code of ethics.
- Providing client information to referral sources as a matter of practice, without first obtaining the client's informed consent to do so.
- When speaking to the media, getting caught up in the moment and sharing information that goes beyond available scientific data.
- Not limiting statements to the media to your own opinions and observations and making statements on behalf of the profession when not authorized to do so.
- Making statements to the media about specific individuals, to include diagnoses, informal assessments, and predictions of future behavior, when you have not personally evaluated that individual.
- Giving specific professional advice to an individual through the media whom you have not comprehensively evaluated.
- Accepting a client's unsolicited offer to provide a testimonial endorsement. Even if offered willingly by the client with no suggestion of it on your part, it may still result in harm to the client and mistrust of your profession by the public.
- In public presentations and advertising, do not present information in a manner intended to stimulate unwarranted anxiety or fear in the audience as a means of stimulating them to seek out your professional services.
- Failing to understand the absence of a barrier between professional and personal uses of social media and the risk of compromised privacy they bring with them.

RELEVANT ETHICS CODE STANDARDS

Public Statements

- AAMFT Code of Ethics (AAMFT, 2012) Principle 3.13, Public Statements, states, "Marriage and family therapists, because of their ability to influence and alter the lives of others, exercise special care when making public their professional recommendations and opinions through testimony and other public statements" (p. 4).

- ACA Code of Ethics (ACA, 2005) Standard C.3.a., Accurate Advertising, states, "When advertising or otherwise representing their services to the public, counselors identify their credentials in an accurate manner that is not false, misleading, deceptive, or fraudulent" (p. 10).
- APA Ethics Code (APA, 2010) Standard 5.01, Avoidance of False or Deceptive Statements, states, "Psychologists do not knowingly make public statements that are false, deceptive or fraudulent" (p. 8). Further, Standard 5.04, Media Presentations, states that when providing "public advice or comment" regardless of the medium used, psychologists "take precautions to ensure that statements are" based on accepted professional knowledge, accurate, and provided in a manner that does "not indicate that a professional relationship has been established with the recipient" (p. 8).
- NASW Code of Ethics (NASW, 2008) Standard, 4.06a, Misrepresentation, states, "Social workers should make clear distinctions between statements made and actions engaged in as a private individual and as a representative of the social work profession, a professional social work organization, or the social workers' employing agency" (p. 7).

Listing Credentials

- AAMFT Code of Ethics (AMFT, 2012) Principle 8.1, Accurate Professional Representation, states, "Marriage and family therapists accurately represent their competencies, education, training, and experience relevant to their practice of marriage and family therapy" (p. 8).
- ACA Code of Ethics (ACA, 2005) Standard C.3.a., Accurate Advertising, states, "When advertising or otherwise representing their services to the public, counselors identify their credentials in an accurate manner that is not false, misleading, deceptive, or fraudulent" (p. 10). Further, Standard C.4.D., Implying Doctoral-Level Competence, states, "Counselors clearly state their highest earned degree in counseling or closely related field. Counselors do not imply doctoral-level competence when only possessing a master's degree in counseling or a related field by referring to themselves as 'Dr.' in a counseling context when their doctorate is not in counseling or related field" (p. 10).
- APA Ethics Code (APA, 2010) Standard 5.01b, Avoidance of False or Deceptive Statements, states, "Psychologists do not make false, deceptive or fraudulent statements concerning…their academic degrees…their credentials" or "their institutional or association affiliations," and Standard 5.01c states, "Psychologists claim degrees as credentials for their health services only if those degrees (1) were earned from a regionally accredited educational institution or (2) were the basis for psychology licensure by the state in which they practice" (p. 8).
- NASW Code of Ethics (NASW, 2008) Standard 4.06c, Misrepresentation, states, "Social workers should ensure that their

representations to clients, agencies, and the public of professional qualifications, credentials, education, competence, affiliations, services provided, or results to be achieved are accurate. Social workers should claim only those relevant professional credentials they actually possess and take steps to correct any inaccuracies or misrepresentations of their credentials by others" (p. 7).

Uninvited Solicitations and Testimonials

- AAMFT Code of Ethics (AAMFT, 2012) Principle 1.3, Multiple Relationships, states, "Marriage and family therapists are aware of their influential positions with respect to clients, and they avoid exploiting the trust and dependency of such persons" (p. 2).
- ACA Code of Ethics (ACA, 2005) Standard C.3.b., Testimonials, states, "Counselors who use testimonials do not solicit them from current clients nor former clients nor any other persons who may be vulnerable to undue influence" (p. 10).
- APA Ethics Code (APA, 2010) Standard 5.06, In-Person Solicitation, states, "Psychologists do not engage, directly or through agents, in uninvited in-person solicitation of business from actual or potential therapy clients/ patients or other persons who because of their particular circumstances are vulnerable to undue influence" (p. 8).
- NASW Code of Ethics (NASW, 2008) states in Standard 4.07b, Solicitations, "Social workers should not engage in uninvited solicitation of potential clients who, because of their circumstances, are vulnerable to undue influence, manipulation, or coercion" (p. 7).

REFERENCES

American Association for Marriage and Family Therapy. (2012). *Code of ethics.* Retrieved from http://www.aamft.org/imis15/content/legal_ethics/code_of_ethics.aspx

American Counseling Association. (2005). *ACA code of ethics.* Retrieved from http://www.counseling.org/Resources/aca-code-of-ethics.pdf

American Psychological Association. (2010). *Ethical principles of psychologists and code of conduct.* Retrieved from http://www.apa.org/ethics

Barnett, J. E., & Klimik, L. (2012). Ethics and business issues in psychology practice. In S. Knapp, M. Gottlieb, M. Handelsman, & L. VandeCreek (Eds.), *APA handbook of ethics in psychology* (Vol. 1, pp. 433–452). Washington, DC: APA Books.

Datillo, F. M., Sadoff, R. L., & Gutheil, T. G. (2003). Board certification in forensic psychiatry and psychology: Separating the chaff from the wheat. *The Journal of Psychiatry and Law, 33*(1), 5–19.

Firestone, R., & Barnett, J. E. (2012). The ethical practice of psychology in rural settings. *The Independent Practitioner, 32,* 102–106.

Kolmes, K. (2012). Social media in the future of professional psychology. *Professional Psychology: Research & Practice, 43,* 606–612.

McGarrah, N. A., Alvord, M. K., Martin, J. N., & Haldeman, D. C. (2009). In the public eye: The ethical practice of media psychology. *Professional Psychology: Research and Practice, 40,* 172–180.

National Association of Social Workers. (2008). *Code of ethics.* Retrieved from http://www.socialworkers.org/pubs/code/code.asp

8

Continuing Professional Development

In the mid-to-late 1970s, when sending graduate students off to clinical practice, professors often gave the advice, "Keep up with your reading." Ordering a few journals and joining a professional book club, as well as going to a professional conference every now and then, was what it took to keep up. Now the amount of information is daunting. The number of journals, books, conferences, and ways information is presented is ever increasing. With the seemingly exponential increase in information each year, one might think, "Why bother, I can't ever keep up." Yet the responsibility of mental health professionals for their professional development is clear, and in some jurisdictions even mandatory for licensure renewal. However, meeting your licensure requirement is not the ultimate goal of professional development.

We believe professional development comes from embracing a commitment to lifelong learning. The goal is to continue one's growth and development far beyond getting one's degree or professional license. You might say, "That is a noble aspiration." We believe it is an imperative. The base of professional knowledge is continually expanding in the form of new information, research findings, and ideas. Furthermore, our clinical competencies can degrade over time. Continuing to update our skills, coupled with the lifelong commitment to our own growth and development, can help us manage the stresses of this work, avoid ethical pitfalls, and provide the best care we possibly can.

READINGS

Mental health professionals do not need to be aware of every piece of information related to their professional activities. In fact, it is possible to be quite competent and to continue to develop as a professional by obtaining information and guidance from quite a few different sources (as discussed hereafter) and not be a walking Library of Congress.

Although the amount of available information is more plentiful than it ever was in the past and can be difficult to sort through, there are ways of streamlining it a bit. Some helpful strategies include:

- Subscribe to the specialty journals that are particularly pertinent to you.
- Join specialty professional associations and subscribe to their publications.
- Set web alerts for content that is relevant to your practice.
- Seek recommendations from other colleagues who have similar practices about the readings that they are finding of use.
- Read abstracts (e.g., PsycSCAN) to assess relevance before delving into the full article.
- Join search services so you can periodically scan for new publications that are most pertinent.
- Subscribe to online journal access services to be able to read journal articles online.

TRAINING

Obtaining training when one is in independent practice is a challenge, yet is important. The key is to make sure that the training obtained is worth the expense (i.e., lost income, lost opportunity, and the cost of attending the training itself). Many training sessions are geared to entry-level professionals in a particular specialty area. It can be difficult to find training at a level that fits within one's own skill set. Moreover, although one can meet licensure requirements from continuing education credits by simply sitting in a training session and filling out the evaluation at its conclusion, the responsibility to truly seek to benefit from the training is important.

There is, in our view, a critical difference between attending continuing education training and seeking a program of specialty training that includes a clinical experiential component with ongoing clinical supervision or consultation. Although continuing education workshops can be a great way to obtain new information, they do not provide the same experience as enrolling in a postgraduate specialty training program that focuses on the development or enhancement of clinical skills or creating new specialty areas.

We recommend seeking training opportunities with an enthusiasm for learning, not to meet some external requirement. If you are investing your time and money, make it worthwhile and commit to the experience.

USE OF LISTSERVS

Listservs (online group e-mail lists) can be a wonderful way of obtaining information and input from colleagues. Some listservs (e.g., Dr. Ken Pope's at www. kspope.com) are announcement-only—broadcast listservs that report on many articles in the professional literature and save you from having to subscribe to many different journals. If you want to read the entire article, you certainly can get that particular reprint. Other listservs are interactive among participants and can provide rapid answers to clinical and ethical questions you may ask. Listservs can also be a very effective way of reducing professional isolation, especially if you select listservs that are well aligned with your specialty area(s).

However, responders on a question-and-answer list are not ultimate authorities on a subject. In fact, many people who respond to questions on a listserv are certain they are offering the correct information, yet it is often only their viewpoint or understanding of the issue. It is important to recognize that on a listserv you are getting the *opinion* of those who respond. There may be many other opinions from other colleagues who are not responding.

Another problem we have experienced with listserv communication is the tendency for some to quickly pull the "It's not ethical" card when someone is approaching a problem or responding to a situation with a client that is contrary to how they would respond in those circumstances. In many cases, ethics is not the issue. Rather there is simply a professional disagreement between the responders. Responders on listservs are not the ultimate authorities on ethical or legal questions. Serious questions of ethical/unethical behavior should be addressed to experts in ethics and law. Many professional organizations have developed ethics hotlines for just this reason. Also, remember that many liability insurance carriers (e.g., American Professional Agency, American Psychological Association Insurance Trust) provide consultation to their insured when a question of ethics or potential civil liability arises.

There can be major issues around confidentiality when it comes to the use of a listserv. When you communicate on a listserv you are making very *public* statements that (unlike speaking in the town square where your comments eventually may evaporate into space) persist indefinitely in cyberspace. It is crucial that you protect any identifying client information if asking for help with a clinical case. Communicating with professionals on a listserv does not mean that the obligations on you around confidentiality are lessened. To the contrary, given that you have no idea who is viewing the posting or how the information is to be used, and your client has not provided informed consent, you need to be extremely careful about what information is posted. This is most salient if you live and work in a small community where even small identifying clues can compromise the confidentiality of the professional relationship. So, for example, a post that reads, "I need input on a case of a dual diagnosis 42-year-old high school teacher" can be problematic if that teacher's brother or cousin is also reading the listserv and sees your posting and your address.

Disclosures on listservs are also not protected. They are not confidential. All postings should be considered part of the public record and should not be conceptualized as a private consultation. Attorneys who are looking to discredit you, or are filing a claim or grievance against you, may use things you say on listservs against you in deposition or at trial. Imagine justifying an approach you took on a case by saying that it was based primarily on what you found on a listserv. This may not be solid footing in which to base an opinion.

PEER CONSULTATION GROUPS

Your work as a mental health professional in private practice can be extremely isolating, especially if you do not work as part of a group practice. There may be little chance to interact with colleagues beyond consulting on a case from time to time. Days can go by with most of your professional interactions being with referral sources and patients. Private practice can be a lonely endeavor. To avoid ethical transgressions, Handelsman (2001) urges clinicians not to practice in isolation. Johnson et al. (2012) support this recommendation, describing how limited our ability to self-assess our competence is and how we must utilize colleagues for consultation and support on an ongoing basis in order to practice competently and ethically.

Creating and participating in a peer consultation group can allow for continuity and professional development throughout the course of your career. A group of professionals who trust one another and have varied and overlapping expertise can offer you a resource that is hard to replicate. These groups can be places to discuss clinical and ethical issues, transference and countertransference, the impact of your work on you and your family, and how to manage the complex demands of clinical practice. The opportunity (with appropriate safeguarding of identifying client information) to obtain diverse perspectives from a group of colleagues can be invaluable. Such groups can also offer emotional support in a safe and non-evaluative environment. Even career planning and business of practice issues can be discussed in these groups.

The input gleaned from a peer supervision group can be specific to the nuances of your situation (unlike what might be offered in a reading of pertinent literature or a formal continuing education course) and can be timely. Such input can also help you address challenges and possibly slippage in skills, which might indicate a need for additional training and mentoring. These needs are often difficult to spot yourself as our own self-assessment may be subject to distortion.

MENTORING

As with peer consultation groups, mentoring provides you with a long-term professional consultative relationship that is tailored to your needs. You can have different mentors over the span of your career, as mentoring is not just for the new graduate or early career professional. Mentoring can have great benefits to both the mentor and the protégé (Johnson, 2002). Mentors can provide a safe and trusting place for you to grow professionally, and can offer you the opportunity for a long-term relationship where you can benefit from the wisdom and views of that colleague, who ideally is a subject matter aspect in your area(s) of specialty.

Mentors can be found in your professional associations, at pertinent professional conferences, and through colleagues. Some professional associations also have mentoring programs.

However, it is important to remember that there is not one body of knowledge or one person who has all the answers to your questions. As a professional you can consult with a mentor, but the responsibility for the clinical work is still your own. This is not the same as the clinical supervision that you obtained prior to licensure. Remember, once you are licensed to practice independently, the input others offer you is exactly that—input. It needs to be incorporated into the full breadth of your best clinical judgment and thought processes.

PERSONAL PSYCHOTHERAPY

One's own personal psychotherapy should not be overlooked as an avenue for professional development. This differs from mentoring, as you may focus on far more personal issues with your psycho therapist than with your mentor. Your psychotherapist may not be a subject matter expert doing similar professional work. However, the insights that develop in psychotherapy based on your own internal processes, reactions to your family of origin, experiences, and reactions to your current life stresses and demands can be invaluable in helping you enhance your responses to the clinical demands you face. Such personal insights can help you avoid taking stances that increase the risk of an ethical lapse. Using your psychotherapy to work through the countertransferences you have in your professional role can be invaluable in helping you respond more effectively to those most difficult patients in your caseload.

It is also important to recognize the challenges and demands of being a mental health clinician. This work can be professionally isolating as well as emotionally demanding. Mental health clinicians experience emotional distress in response to the clinical work we do with clients (Baker, 2003). In fact, if we do not adequately address the ongoing stressors of our work, this can lead to the development of symptoms of burnout, which can easily degrade our clinical competence and effectiveness (Rupert & Morgan, 2005). Further, clinicians who treat clients suffering from various forms of trauma may find themselves traumatized by this experience themselves, experiencing what Figley (1995) has termed *compassion fatigue*, also known as *vicarious traumatization*.

Beyond all these work-related factors, we each must cope with and manage our personal lives and all the stressors related to them. Although we might like to think that we can leave work at the office and keep our personal lives from affecting our professional work, research clearly demonstrates how our professional and personal lives interact, affecting and influencing each other (Pipes, Holstein, & Aguirre, 2005). Thus, we recommend that each mental health clinician consider personal psychotherapy at various points in their careers to help ensure competent, ethical, and effective practice.

THE ROLE OF SELF-CARE, BURNOUT PREVENTION, AND THE PROMOTION OF WELLNESS

There is an old expression that speaks to when you put your foot in the river: The river is never the same. The expression goes on to state that neither is the foot. The work of the mental health professional is difficult. As just noted, we can experience the vicarious trauma of the people who we help and who have been injured by accident, by intention, or by evil. There is an intensity, level of focus, and responsibility of this work that can be life saving from a literal and psychological standpoint. At the same time, we are not immune to the struggles and challenges of our clients, our own lives, and those of the people we love. Although we change the river, the river changes us.

O'Connor (2001) summarizes research on the incidence of distress, burnout, and problems with professional competence experienced by practicing mental health professionals. The data clearly point to the findings that despite the fact that we are mental health professionals, we are not immune from experiencing life's trials and tribulations. We experience the same difficulties others do: substance abuse, depression, health concerns, relationship difficulties, financial stresses, and loneliness. Barnett and Cooper (2009) advocate for creating a culture of self-care for practicing mental health professionals, including the suggestion of mandatory continuing education to highlight the importance of this area. Norcross and Guy (2007) suggest that self-care should be an ongoing preventive activity for all mental health professionals as a way of taking care of themselves, but also being more effective with those that clinicians serve.

To function effectively, we need to make sure that we are taking good care of ourselves. There is not one size that fits all. There is not even one size that might fit you for the long run. Rather, you are likely to have different needs and require different outlets and supports throughout the course of your career. Be sure to make time to address your own personal needs, whether it is through time with family and friends, exercise, play, intellectual pursuits, hobbies, attending to your spiritual side, or a combination of the above.

At times there can be great demand for your services. This demand can outstrip the time available. Be sure to invest in taking care of yourself. Such care is likely to help you be more effective with others and avoid those ethical lapses we have so often spoken about in this book.

The essential point here is to make sure you are routinely practicing self-care in an intentional way. We need to actively work to maintain wellness and balance in our own lives. Without doing so, the distress we experience will likely lead to burnout and related problems with professional competence, often contributing to the risk of unethical decisions and actions. Routinely engage in an ongoing program of self-care and wellness promotion that is integrated into your ongoing lifestyle and addresses the physical, emotional, relationship, and spiritual aspects of your life—yes, *your* life (not just those who you try to help).

We are also not immune from experiencing physical illness that may impair our ability to practice. Johnson and Barnett (2011) describe reasons why psychologists may choose to continue to practice even when they are gravely ill. Some of these reasons include a love of the work, genuine caring for the client, and economic fears about loss of income and maintaining the viability of a practice. These authors suggest that due to self-assessment bias these individuals may not be in the best position to adequately determine what is in the best interest of their clients. In such circumstances they provide a number of recommendations for the clinician to consider in response to the medical crisis and the ability to practice, recommendations for how colleagues could respond, and how credentialing and regulatory boards could respond.

STAYING AWARE OF LOCAL LAWS, REGULATIONS, AND CHANGES

It is easy to miss something crucial. Laws and regulations affecting your practice come in many different shapes and sizes. Tax law, employment law, statutes on confidentiality, Medicare regulations, patients' bills of rights, and of course overarching health care acts all can impact your practice. It is far too easy to miss something by simply watching the news, going online or listening to the radio. As we've heard for decades, "Ignorance of the law is no excuse." Our ethical codes require us to obey the law, yet it is far too easy to miss what is happening when key language may be hidden in, for example, a "transportation bill." That is where our professional associations come into play. They often will have the latest information about the status of proposed and approved legislation and its impact on your practice. Your dues help support their initiatives and help you keep current on this information. Seek and stay attuned to what is current and relevant.

ETHICAL CHALLENGES

- Wanting to run from the need to continue one's professional development as a result of being overwhelmed by the plethora of available information.
- Avoiding unintended confidential disclosures on listservs and in other communications with professionals not involved on a case.
- Competencies can erode over time. This erosion may be outside of our own awareness.
- It is difficult to keep up with the new research that informs your practice and is continually being made available.
- Finding the time to practice self-care and promote our own wellness on a regular ongoing basis.
- Attending to the effects of being a mental health clinician on our own wellness and clinical effectiveness and knowing when to seek consultation, support, and assistance.

KEY POINTS TO KEEP IN MIND

- Your professional skills can deteriorate over time. You may not notice this change for the worse.
- It is important to stay up to date with new developments and research in your specialty area(s).
- Listservs are not confidential environments.
- You ultimately are responsible for the care you provide. Use the input from colleagues to help you shape, but not direct, your decision making.
- This work is difficult, and although you affect the people you work with, the work (and the people) can affect you.
- Use other professionals to provide input about potential areas for skill building. Mentors, peer support groups, and your own psychotherapy can be invaluable.
- The prevention of difficulties through ongoing self-care and wellness promotion is far superior to responding to symptoms of burnout and vicarious traumatization after they develop.

PRACTICAL RECOMMENDATIONS

- Keep all identifying information off of listserv postings. Use the telephone or e-mail backchannel to a specific individual if you are seeking more personal and specific discussions.
- Incorporate clinical input from colleagues into your own thinking about your work, but do not rely on it as the definitive direction.
- Create a constellation of competence (Johnson et al., 2012) that may include friends, colleagues, mentors, a peer support group, clinical supervision, and the like, to help promote your ongoing wellness, competence, and ethical practice.
- Document all consultations you receive about ethical dilemmas.
- Join your professional associations (state, national, and specialty), read their updates on laws and regulations and make use of their support services.
- Be sure to address your needs for support, rest, and self-care.
- Be careful to make sure you avoid professional isolation.

PITFALLS TO AVOID

- Giving up on professional development because one is overwhelmed by the amount of available information.
- Assuming the *opinions* of others on a listserv represent clear and accepted standards around ethics or clinical direction.

- Professional isolation.
- Relying on your own assessment of your competence, training needs, and ethical decision making, without seeking input from respected and trusted colleagues.
- Violating confidentiality on listservs.
- Assuming your comments on listservs are not public.
- Seeing yourself as a "helper" but neglecting to help yourself.

RELEVANT ETHICS CODE STANDARDS

Maintaining Awareness of Legal Regulations and Statutes.

- AAMFT Code of Ethics (AAMFT, 2012) Principle 3.2, Knowledge of Regulatory Standards, states, "Marriage and family therapists maintain adequate knowledge of and adhere to applicable laws, ethics, and professional standards" (p. 4).
- ACA Code of Ethics (ACA, 2005) Standard C.1., Knowledge of Standards, states, "Counselors have a responsibility to read, understand, and follow the *ACA Code of Ethics* and adhere to applicable laws and regulations" (p. 9).
- APA Ethics Code (APA, 2010) Standard 1.02, Conflicts Between Ethics and Law, Regulations, or Other Governing Legal Authority, states, "If psychologists' ethical responsibilities conflict with law, regulations or other governing legal authority, psychologists clarify the nature of the conflict, make known their commitment to the Ethics Code and take reasonable steps to resolve the conflict consistent with the General Principles and Ethical Standards of the Ethics Code. Under no circumstances may this standard be used to justify or defend violating human rights" (p. 4).
- NASW Code of Ethics (NASW, 2008) Preamble states, "In addition to this *Code,* there are many other sources of information about ethical thinking that may be useful. Social workers should consider ethical theory and principles generally, social work theory and research, laws, regulations, agency policies, and other relevant codes of ethics, recognizing that among codes of ethics social workers should consider the *NASW Code of Ethics* as their primary source" (p. 1).

Maintaining Competence

- AAMFT Code of Ethics (AAMFT, 2012) Principle 3.1, Maintenance of Competency, states, "Marriage and family therapists pursue knowledge of new developments and maintain their competence in marriage and family therapy through education, training, or supervised experience" (p. 3).

- ACA Code of Ethics (ACA, 2005) Standard C.2.f., Continuing Education, states, "Counselors recognize the need for continuing education to acquire and maintain a reasonable level of awareness of current scientific and professional information in their fields of activity. They take steps to maintain competence in the skills they use" (p. 9).
- APA Ethics Code (APA, 2010) Standard 2.03, Maintaining Competence, states, "Psychologists undertake ongoing efforts to develop and maintain their competence" (p. 5).
- NASW Code of Ethics (NASW, 2008) Standard 1.04b, Competence, states, "Social workers should provide services in substantive areas or use intervention techniques or approaches that are new to them only after engaging in appropriate study, training, consultation, and supervision from people who are competent in those interventions or techniques" (p. 2).

Personal Problems and Conflicts

- AAMFT Code of Ethics (AAMFT, 2012) Principle 3.3, Seek Assistance, states, "Marriage and family therapists seek appropriate professional assistance for their personal problems or conflicts that may impair work performance or clinical judgment" (p. 4).
- ACA Code of Ethics (ACA, 2005) Standard C.2.g., Impairment, states, "Counselors are alert to the signs of impairment from their own physical, mental, or emotional problems and refrain from offering or providing professional services when such impairment is likely to harm a client or others. They seek assistance for problems that reach the level of professional impairment, and, if necessary, they limit, suspend, or terminate their professional responsibilities until such time it is determined that they may safely resume their work" (p. 9).
- APA Ethics Code (APA, 2010) Standard 2.06, Personal Problems and Conflicts, states, "(a) Psychologists refrain from initiating an activity when they know or should know that there is a substantial likelihood that their personal problems will prevent them from performing their work-related activities in a competent manner. (b) When psychologists become aware of personal problems that may interfere with their performing work-related duties adequately, they take appropriate measures, such as obtaining professional consultation or assistance and determine whether they should limit, suspend or terminate their work-related duties" (p. 5).
- NASW Code of Ethics (NASW, 2008) Standard 4.05, Impairment, states, "Social workers whose personal problems, psychosocial distress, legal problems, substance abuse, or mental health difficulties interfere with their professional judgment and performance should immediately seek consultation and take appropriate remedial action by seeking professional help, making adjustments in workload, terminating practice, or taking any other steps necessary to protect clients and others" (p. 7).

REFERENCES

American Association for Marriage and Family Therapy. (2012). *Code of ethics.* Retrieved from http://www.aamft.org/imis15/content/legal_ethics/code_of_ethics.aspx

American Counseling Association. (2005). *ACA code of ethics.* Retrieved from http://www.counseling.org/Resources/aca-code-of-ethics.pdf

American Psychological Association. (2010). *Ethical principles of psychologists and code of conduct.* Retrieved from http://www.apa.org/ethics

Baker, E. K. (2003). *Caring for ourselves: A therapist's guide to personal and professional well-being.* Washington, DC: American Psychological Association.

Barnett, J. E., & Cooper, N. (2009). Creating a culture of self-care. *Clinical Psychology: Science and Practice, 16*(1), 16–20.

Figley, C. R. (1995). *Compassion fatigue: Secondary traumatic stress from treating the traumatized.* New York: Brunner/Mazel.

Handelsman, M. (2001). Learning to become ethical. In S. Walfish & A. K. Hess (Eds.), *Succeeding in graduate school: The career guide for the psychology student* (pp. 189–202). Mahwah, NJ: Erlbaum.

Johnson, W. B., (2002). The intentional mentor: Strategies and guidelines for the practice of mentoring. *Professional Psychology: Research and Practice, 33*, 88–96.

Johnson, W. B., & Barnett, J. E. (2011). Preventing problems of professional competence in the face of life-threatening illness. *Professional Psychology: Research and Practice, 42*, 285–293.

Johnson, W. B., Barnett, J. E., Elman, N., Forrest, L., & Kaslow, N. J. (2012). The competent community: Toward a radical reformulation of professional ethics. *American Psychologist, 67*, 557–569.

National Association of Social Workers. (2008). *Code of ethics.* Retrieved from http://www.socialworkers.org/pubs/code/code.asp

Norcross, J. C., & Guy, J. D. (2007). *Leaving it at the office.* New York, NY: Guilford Press.

O'Connor, M. F. (2001). On the etiology and effective management of professional distress and impairment among psychologists. *Professional Psychology: Research and Practice, 32*(4), 345–350.

Pipes, R. B., Holstein, J. E., & Aguirre, M. G. (2005). Examining the personal-professional distinction: Ethics codes and the difficulty of drawing a boundary. *American Psychologist, 60*, 325–334.

Rupert, P. A., & Morgan, D. J. (2005). Work setting and burnout among professional psychologists. *Professional Psychology: Research and Practice, 36*, 544–550.

9

Leaving a Practice

All good things must come to an end. Many people decide to leave their practice. It may be because they have been in practice for 30 to 40 years and have determined that it is time to retire. It may be because the clinician tried private practice as a career path but found they preferred to use their skill set in an organizational or educational setting. It may be because it is time for a geographical change for personal reasons, or it may be due to illness and no longer being able to work.

Regardless of the reason for leaving a practice, private practitioners must address ethical issues before they close the doors. One cannot simply wake up one morning and decide that they no longer want to be in practice, place a sign on the door that says, "I am now retired. Best of luck to you," and then never be heard from again. Although private practitioners are small business owners, the provision of mental health services is not similar to owning a restaurant or clothing store, where one can indeed put up such a sign and the only ramification is a few disappointed customers. As licensed health care providers we have obligations to those we serve and have served. Barnett (1997) notes that failure to adequately plan how one will leave a practice may "have a negative impact on our patients, create a significant liability risk, or lead to ill feelings between former patients" (p. 181).

There are many issues to consider when closing a practice that we will highlight in this chapter. These include (a) notification to the group where one practices, if one is not a sole proprietor, (b) developing an exit strategy in telling clients that you will no longer be practicing, (c) ensuring continuity of care for your clients, (d) maintenance of records, (e) selling a practice, and (f) malpractice insurance into retirement.

NOTIFYING YOUR GROUP THAT YOU ARE LEAVING THE PRACTICE

Most clinicians are so happy to join a practice that they rarely pay attention to the details to which they become contractually bound when they decide to leave it. Most contracts that clinicians sign when they join a practice contain a clause about a time frame for providing notice that they will be leaving the practice. Contract notification time periods mostly range from 30 to 90 days; however, we have seen contracts with time frames as long as 6 to 12 months. We have also seen contracts where it is the clinician's responsibility to find a replacement for them that is acceptable to the group. By including such language in the contract, the practice owners are trying to protect their income, but we would never advocate signing a contract with such a clause.

In considering leaving a practice, it is important that the clinician pay careful attention to the details listed in the contract. Of course, just as with your contracts with MCOs, the best time to pay attention to the details is *before* you sign the contract. For example, the contract should contain language regarding ownership of records. If the organizational structure is one of a clinic or a group practice, the records may belong to them, rather than the individual practitioner. Copying some or all of the records would require obtaining informed consent from the patient or responsible party. On the other hand, if the arrangement is that of a sole proprietor clinician who is renting or sharing space and services, then the records should belong to the clinician and should leave with them.

The contract should also describe a protocol for how former or future clients can contact the clinician who is leaving the practice. This may not be an issue if the decision to leave is done under amicable terms. However, if there is animosity between the parties, clients should not be made to suffer or be inconvenienced by being placed in the middle of the dispute. Former clients have a right to be able to contact their former clinician to resume counseling, obtain records, or consult with them for any reason they like. It would be a disservice to clients to call a practice and ask to speak to Dr. C, and be told that she had left the practice and left no forwarding address or telephone number, when in fact that information was readily available to be communicated to the caller. Clinicians should negotiate their potential exit from the practice in the contract they sign to join it. As part of their exit, clinicians should ask to maintain a voice mail box they can check for a specified amount of time (we recommend 90 days). They should also ask that if a client calls to speak with them to schedule an appointment, that their forwarding contact information be provided to the caller. It would be exploitation of the client calling to schedule an appointment with Dr. C only to be told, "Dr. C is no longer with us, but Dr. D is now with our practice and you may schedule an appointment with her."

Similarly, there should be language in the agreement that neither you nor the practice group will be speak negatively of each other or disclose the circumstances of the departure to others. This can help reduce the likelihood that your old practice will demean you to the referral community.

TELLING CLIENTS THAT YOU WILL NO LONGER BE PRACTICING

Having closed practices in the past, we will tell you that having a conversation with a client to inform them that you will no longer be their psychotherapist is extremely difficult. If there is a strong therapeutic alliance, both the client and clinician will be experiencing a loss. For clients this can result in significant transference reactions, especially if they have a history of abandonment or difficulty with attachment. For the psychotherapist this can prompt countertransference issues if they have concerns about being viewed as the person who is causing the emotional pain, as well as financial fears that the client may decide to terminate sooner than the clinician had planned. These clinical issues must be addressed with sensitivity and skill, and the wise psychotherapist will consult with a colleague regarding staying centered when dealing with the termination with so many clients at the same time.

Koocher (2003) advises that "thoughtful planning offers the best strategy for avoiding ethical problems associated with practice transition" (p. 386). If the closing of the practice is voluntary and not for emergency reasons, the clinician is typically aware of a planned end date. As opposed to a restaurant or hardware store, the provision of mental health services must take into consideration several issues that should be guided by ethical principles. Careful planning must be done that takes into consideration the needs of clients, as opposed to the needs of the clinician, especially the need to continue to earn a living.

In discussing practice relocation, Manosevitz and Hays (2003) state, "A date must be set after which new referrals will not be accepted" (p. 337). If the clinician is not yet ready to announce the closing of their practice, simply stating "I'm not accepting new clients at this time" may suffice. This date may depend upon the clinician's type of practice. For example, it may be different if one practices long-term insight-oriented psychotherapy, versus short-term cognitive therapy for anxiety or depression. If one generally does practice short-term psychotherapy, it will be important to reassess each client's treatment needs after a few sessions to ensure that they are not actually going to need long-term treatment. If they do, it becomes imperative that the clinician have a discussion with the client about their intention to close the practice. At this time it is likely in the client's best interest to refer to a clinician who can help them reach their long-term goals.

The next task in the process is to decide when to tell clients. Manosevitz and Hays (2003) suggest that "deciding whom to tell and when could be determined by treatment orientation, perceptions of a patient's need to know and process, and frequency of contact" (p. 377). They also suggest that it is important to create enough time for the patient to process the emotional issues of the clinician leaving. Unfortunately there is no blueprint or formula for determining a specific time frame, and no one time frame will work uniformly for all of the clients in the clinician's practice. Zuckerman (2008) suggests that clients "must be given sufficient time to make the best resolutions and least traumatic alternative arrangements" (p. 36). At a minimum, practitioners should consider the length of the client's treatment, the nature of the treatment relationship, any history of dependency or abandonment issues, and the client's current treatment needs, when deciding how much notice to give and when and how to initiate and carry out this discussion.

McGee (2003) advises that subsequent to discussing the practice closure with a client, documentation of this discussion should be included in the treatment record. We have had the experience of a client becoming emotionally distraught when being told of the closure of a practice, only to be contacted eight months later about an administrative issue and their stating, "Yes, I heard something about you moving back East." This reinforces McGee's point, as termination has the possibility of being an emotionally charged event for the client and may interfere with information processing and retention.

While setting separate dates to tell each client may be a clinical ideal, on a practical basis this may create a firestorm for the practitioner. Bennett et al. (2006) suggest that in small communities it may be wise to set one specific date and to inform all of your clients around the same time. Their rationale for this is that in such communities, the news of the closing of a practice may spread quickly. Although it may be impossible to avoid, clients have the right to hear that the psychotherapy relationship will be ending from their psychotherapist directly and not from a friend or neighbor. Bennett et al. suggest applying this principle in small communities, but we would extend the idea of picking a date and informing clients around the same time to communities of all sizes. There are too many "small world" experiences and it is best if the client hears this information directly in the context of a psychotherapy session.

In addition to current clients, there is also the issue of informing former clients that the practice is closing. There are no clear guidelines for which former clients to inform. Bennett et al. (2006) suggest using clinical judgment in deciding, noting, "Some patients will appreciate knowing your decision, and it may help them avoid inconvenience and emotional upset if they feel they need additional services and always thought that you would be available" (p. 215). We suggest that a conservative approach would be for the clinician to mail letters to each of their clients for the past two years, letting them know that the practice will be closing. Zuckerman (2008) suggests that the letter announcing the closing include "why you are closing up shop; exactly when the office will close; who will have your records and how to reach them; whom clients can call in an emergency, and what other therapists or community resources are available if they want more services" (p. 36). Clients may ask for a recommendation of another clinician should they want to continue in psychotherapy at a later date. You may consider providing a few names of trusted colleagues as potential referral sources in the future, or sharing information with them about a referral network or directory, such as those generally available through the websites of professional organizations. McGee (2003) also suggests that copies of any letters sent to current or former clients about the practice closure be placed in the client's treatment record. Zuckerman (2008) recommends sending a copy of the termination letter to your licensing board, so they will be aware that you closed your practice and who will have custody of your records.

We will also point out there may be regulatory requirements regarding the closure of your practice. For example, in one state a clinician must place an advertisement in the public notices classified section of the local newspaper regarding the closure of the practice for at least 30 days. This advertisement must indicate the date of closing and how any interested parties may obtain their treatment records should they desire to access them in the future. Thus, it is important to carefully read your jurisdiction's laws and regulations regarding independent practice for any special requirements.

Earlier we discussed issues related to signing a restrictive covenant (e.g., non-competition clause) when the clinician is asked to join a practice. If the clinician has signed such a clause it is imperative that they review it carefully prior to leaving the practice, and prior to informing their clients, referral partners, or the group practice. It may be important to consider the ethical implications of what might subsequently ensue, especially as it relates to referral recommendations to clients. Some restrictive covenants essentially imply that the "client belongs to the practice" and not to the clinician. The practice may decide to divide the caseload equally among the other clinicians in the office, regardless of specific client needs. For example, if a client's clinician specializes in a specific area (e.g., personality disorders, social skills training with children) and the other clinicians in the practice do not share the same specialty skills, then it would not be in the client's best interests to continue care with someone within the practice, if outside local experts are available. Under such conditions we strongly suggest that the clinician advocate for their clients with the practice group, but understand they have contractual obligations that may conflict with ethical obligations. Barnett (1997) suggests the possibility that conflicts over such issues could possibly be resolved through mediation or consultation with an ethics committee or licensing board, noting that "regardless of contractual obligations or issues, each patient's welfare remains the paramount consideration which should guide all deliberations and decisions" (p. 195).

ENSURING CONTINUITY OF CARE

When closing their practice, clinicians may just not close their doors and let clients fend for themselves. We must attend to our clients' ongoing needs and remain cognizant of our ongoing obligations to promote their best interests. Accordingly, when clinicians inform clients that they will be closing their practice at some future date, decisions must be made regarding future treatment needs. Regarding continuity of care, Barnett (1997) states, "It seems clear that the legal and ethical burden rests squarely on the provider's shoulders to focus on the patient's treatment needs and to take all reasonable steps to ensure that these needs are met" (p. 183). These decisions should focus on both short-term and long-term treatment planning.

The mental health professions' focus on autonomous decision making suggests that clients should be able to participate in this treatment planning process. For example, if Dr. D tells Ms. Doe that she will be closing her practice in 6 months, Dr. D may prefer to work with her the entire time to (a) continue working on the issues that have been the focus of psychotherapy, (b) work through termination issues, (c) make a smooth transition to a new treating clinician, and (d) maintain her income. However, Ms. Doe may prefer other plans. This might include but not be limited to (a) increasing the frequency of sessions to several times per week, so maximal focus may be placed on the clinical issues being addressed; (b) decreasing the frequency of sessions so that attachment to Dr. D may be lessened over time, assisting Ms. Doe in transitioning to more independent functioning; or (c) stopping psychotherapy almost immediately and transferring to another psychotherapist—they are eventually going to have to transition, so why not do so now? Regardless of what course is chosen, respect for our clients is demonstrated by having them be part of the decision-making process through open discussion of these issues, to include the client's needs and preferences. Clinicians need to be especially mindful of the possible countertransference issue of money, as they cannot let their economic needs (and therefore having the conscious or unconscious need for the client to remain involved in treatment for a time frame that meets the clinician's needs, rather than the clinical needs of the client) interfere with autonomous decision making by clients.

If the clinician refers the client to another practitioner for further care, the client should be asked if they would like the two professionals to communicate with each other. With appropriate written permission from the client, Barnett (1997) suggests providing copies of assessment and treatment records to the new clinician, as well as a transfer note or summary.

In the case of relocation (and not retirement), Manosevitz and Hays (2003) discuss the possibility of a psychotherapist continuing with a client via telephone sessions. The decision to do so should be made on an individual basis and within ethical and regulatory standards, and in compliance with APA's Guidelines for the Practice of Telepsychology (available at http://www.apapracticecentral.org/update/2013/10-24/telepsychology-review.aspx). For example, if the clinician moves to another jurisdiction, and they want to continue with a client via telephone sessions or secure videoconferencing, it is essential that they retain their license to practice in the jurisdiction where the client resides. If not, they may be considered to be practicing in the client's jurisdiction without a professional license. If the sessions are conducted via videoconferencing, it is essential that that medium in which the sessions are conducted is compliant with HIPAA guidelines. The decision to continue must be made with the best interests of the client in mind, and not the need for the clinician to have continued income while they are building a practice in their new location. Discussion of ethics standards for providing services across distances utilizing various technologies may be found in Harris and Younggren (2012). These authors point to the need for each clinician to do a risk–benefit analysis as to whether this alternative form of communication serves the best interests of the client, and to ensure that its use is consistent with the client's ongoing treatment needs. They suggest being especially cautious in providing such services when the client has significant psychological difficulties, such as an acting out diagnosis or risk for self-harm. Harris and Younggren (2012) also point to the need for the clinician to be (a) competent and proficient in delivering electronic services, and (b) cognizant of which laws regarding confidentiality and record keeping apply when delivering services remotely, whether it be the jurisdiction where the client resides or where the clinician resides.

INFORMING REFERRAL PARTNERS

There is no ethics standard to suggest that a clinician closing their practice has to inform their referral partners regarding this transition. However, we think it is common courtesy for the clinician to let them know that they will no longer be serving as a referral partner. Indeed, if there has been a long-standing relationship, the referral partner has likely come to count on the clinician to be there to meet the mental health needs of those they serve.

The clinician may be seeing clients for which there is third party oversight of the clients' treatment progress. Such examples may include clients who are on probation or parole, or those who were supervisory referrals by an employee assistance program, or in cases where a health care provider has been found to be impaired but is in a supervised monitoring program sanctioned by a licensing board. In these instances it is essential that the clinician leaving their practice coordinate continuing care arrangements for the client with the referral partner. These particular clients may be limited in their ability to choose a provider to one that is approved by this third party. Clinicians who work closely with the court system should also inform their contacts in that system so the court is not ordering people into treatment or for evaluation when the clinician is no longer available. For this reason, it is in the client's best interest for the clinician to inform the referral partner they will be closing their practice and to consult with them regarding the most appropriate subsequent provider that can meet both the therapeutic needs of the client, and the administrative needs of the third party. These should be done well in advance of closing one's practice so that there is ample time to taking those steps that serve the client's best interests.

The clinician also may have contracts to provide services for partners in the community. Each of these contracts likely contains provisions regarding termination of the agreement. These should be carefully reviewed as part of the planning process of closing the practice, as the clinician may be obligated to provide (a) services until a certain date, (b) a certain amount of notice before terminating the contract (e.g., 90 days), or (c) sufficient time to the partners to find a new clinician.

MAINTENANCE OF RECORDS

Ethics codes in the mental health professions address the issue of what happens to a client's records when the private practitioner closes their practice. Zuckerman (2008) indicates several reasons why records should be preserved, including (a) complying with laws and ethics, (b) assuring continuity of care for clients, (c) defending yourself from a belated accusation, and (d) qualifying a client for some service or benefits in the future. Clients may begin psychotherapy and want their new clinician to review their previous records. Zuckerman notes that in malpractice cases the statute of limitations may refer to a certain time period that begins when a client "has discovered their damage" (p. 34). That is, although the client may have been seen 10 years ago, they may have only learned of their damage in the past year. Thus, although a long time has passed, the client's treatment record may be crucial in defending yourself against charges of unethical behavior, negligence, or malpractice. For this reason Zuckerman actually suggests retaining adult treatment records for at least 12 years beyond termination of services (regardless of local statutes), or keeping a written summary of each patient's treatment forever. Clients may also seek out benefits of some type (e.g., Social Security disability, accommodation in a learning situation, a workers compensation claim, or personal injury following the experience of a traumatic event), and these records may be crucial data in determining their eligibility to receive these benefits. From a practical standpoint, whereas in the past keeping dated records could require unending amounts of storage space and locked cabinets, it is now possible to scan each record and secure vast amounts of files in a relatively small space. Consequently, we recommend that you store old records indefinitely.

In addition to ethics codes, the issue of records also falls into the regulatory arena. Licensing law statutes discuss requirements for record retention by the private practitioner. These requirements vary by jurisdiction. For example, in Georgia records must remain accessible to an adult client for 7 years from the last date of service. For minors, these records must be accessible for a minimum of 7 years beyond when they reach majority. So, if the child was evaluated at age 4, these records must be accessible until they are 25 years old.

Private practitioners may choose to be their own records custodian. That is, they retain custody of the records, and whenever requests come in for copies of the records, they honor them. As part of their professional will, the practitioner must make alternative arrangements in cases where they are not able to honor the request due to being incapacitated or deceased. Bennett et al. (2006) describe how an estate can be sued for malpractice if records retention or management are done improperly. That is, even though the clinician is deceased, someone must properly be responsible for the client records. The clinician should make arrangements with a professional versed in mental health ethics and law to serve in the role of records custodian, and not simply leave the task to a family member who is not in the profession. It is also important to notify all current and former clients of the existence of this custodian of records and how to access the records. For example, in the aforementioned notice placed in a local newspaper, the identity of the records custodian would be included, as well as this professional's contact information for requesting any needed copies.

Prior to a clinician's taking action to dispose of former patients' treatment records, Barnett (1997) advocates for consultation with an attorney regarding state law concerning such disposal. He notes, "Several states have specific requirements for former patients to be notified in writing that their records will be destroyed, on what date, and how the record or a summary may be obtained prior to that date" (p. 186).

SELLING A PRACTICE

It is extremely difficult to sell a mental health practice. This is especially the case if one is a solo practitioner. In such instances, unless the clinician can transfer preexisting contracts for services or consultations, the primary value of the practice is the solo practitioner him- or herself. In Walfish and Barnett (2009), Henry Harlow describes ways to position a practice that will be attractive to a potential buyer. This includes building a "systems-based" practice rather than one particular individual's "personality-based" practice, and having a transition period where the buyer can seamlessly take over the practice from the seller. An example of such a transition is presented in Weitz and Samuels (1990). In this instance Weitz sold his practice to Samuels, but there was a significant overlap and transition time before Weitz left the practice completely. Samuels was integrated into the practice and introduced to referral partners. Over time it changed from being a practice solely identified with Weitz to one identified with Samuels.

Ethics issues must be taken into consideration if one is to sell a practice. These revolve around the general issues of maintaining confidentiality of current and past clients, and not being exploitive of clients for the personal gain of the seller.

A clinician cannot simply "sell" their current or past clients to a potential buyer. Woody (1997) points out that "transfer of ownership of a psychological practice requires special protection of client lists and records" (p. 78). Koocher (2003) notes that the selling clinician must ask each client for consent to share his or her records with the potential buyer of the practice. A client would have to give permission to the owner of the practice to discuss their case, for the potential buyer to look at their records, or even to know their name. Permission to provide client names and records to a third party must come as written permission from each client. (An exception to this would be if the clinician had made arrangements for someone to be custodian of their records in case of incapacitation or death).

Clinician A therefore cannot simply announce to his current and past clients that Clinician B is taking over their practice, and if they would like to continue care (or return to care), to simply contact Clinician B to make an appointment either now or at some point in the future should they be in need of services. The transfer of all of Clinician A's clients to Clinician B has the potential to be exploitive of the clients for the financial benefits of the clinicians involved in the sale. Each client retains the right to decide whom he or she would like to work with in psychotherapy (including a mental health professional not associated with your practice). Further, it is possible that the clinician who purchases your practice does not possess identical clinical competencies to yours. It is unlikely that this new clinician is the appropriate professional to work with every one of your clients. As it relates to selling a practice, it is each mental health clinician's primary

responsibility to ensure that our actions are motivated by a commitment to benefitting our clients, and not our personal gain.

Walfish and Zimmerman (2013) suggest that each referral a clinician makes to
another professional has to be made with the best interests of the client in mind,
and not be motivated by the best interests of the clinicians involved. Each client
that moves from the care of Clinician A to Clinician B must be considered an
individual referral. When there is money involved in the sale of the practice, it
may be difficult for the clinician to be objective and indeed not create a conflict
of interest that they ethically aspire to avoid. Under ideal conditions a neutral
third-party clinician would review each case and provide guidance as to whether
or not it is appropriate for the client to be transferred to Clinician B.

In addition to Clinician A making the referral, it is also the responsibility of
Clinician B to make a determination if they should accept the referral. This decision should be based on their clinical expertise, and not on a mindset that says,
"This client comes with the sale of the practice, so therefore I should be able to see
them." If the practice primarily focuses on a specialized niche area (e.g., ADHD
evaluation, eating disorders, dialectical behavior therapy for borderline personality disorder), then a transfer of most clients may be justified assuming Clinician
B shares Clinician A's skill set. However, if the practice is a more generalized one
in which Clinician A treated clients with a wide variety of clinical problem areas,
then Clinician B runs the risk of accepting clients into treatment that fall outside
of her or his areas of expertise.

MALPRACTICE INSURANCE INTO RETIREMENT

There are two types of malpractice insurance for mental health providers. The
first type, "claims-made," only provides coverage while the policy is in effect. If
you end coverage for any reason, the coverage ceases. For example, if the policy
was in effect in 2012 and you discontinued the coverage in 2013, the insurance
would not cover a claim made against you in 2014 for alleged malpractice that
took place in 2012. The second type, "occurrence," is the type of policy where
coverage never ceases. Using our example, with occurrence you would still have
malpractice insurance coverage in place in 2014, even though you had stopped
the policy in 2013.

The reason this is important is that clients can make claims against your previous professional behavior even after you have retired and are no longer practicing.
For those who have occurrence insurance this is not an issue, because malpractice
coverage is in place for life. For those who had claims-made coverage, we advise
that a "tail" be purchased to ensure continued coverage, because a significant
portion of negligence claims will be made years after the alleged event (Bennett
et al., 2006).

Bennett et al. (2006) point out that many mental health professionals continue
to provide some type of professional service even after they have formally retired
from their full-time job. This may come in the form of part-time clinical practice,

providing consultation or clinical supervision to unlicensed or junior-level professionals, or even doing pro bono clinical work at a charitable organization. Bennett et al. note that these indirect service roles, or providing direct services for fewer hours per month than prior to retirement, is still accompanied by professional responsibility (and liability risk). We think that as long as one is providing any professional services, the possibility of a malpractice suit exists. Therefore, we suggest that mental health professionals either continue their malpractice coverage if they are going to be providing professional services of any type (including in a charitable organization), or not provide any services at all.

Bennett et al. (2006) also warn about informally practicing when in retirement. They present the example of the seemingly innocuous behavior of providing a former client with a referral to another clinician. Noting that mental health clinicians have been sued for providing "improper referrals," they recommend against providing such referrals. Rather, they suggest the client should be advised to contact one of their physicians, their insurance carrier, or a local professional organization that provides a referral service. Clearly this is a conservative approach, but they are correct when they opine that if something goes wrong, that the well-intentioned clinician can be sued for "improper referral."

THE PROFESSIONAL PRACTICE WILL

The preceding discussion assumes that closing a practice is a conscious and planned choice of the mental health clinician. No practitioner likes to think about their own possible incapacitation or death. However, because clinicians serve the public, and clients' best interests are paramount, our ethics codes require that we do have safeguards in place should either of these occur.

The term for the document that describes what should take place should the clinician become incapacitated or die is a *professional will.* Although not a legal document, it does express the directions of the clinician for what is to take place on behalf of their clients' interests when they are no longer able to perform certain services or provide information. In addition to meeting legal and ethical obligations, Ballard (2005) points to the importance of having such a document to ensure that the task of fulfilling this role does not fall to a family member. As family members are not usually licensed mental health professionals, they should not be expected to know how to comply with legal and ethical requirements that are still in place, even though the clinician may have passed on.

Zuckerman (2008) notes that no official guidelines exist for what should be contained in a professional will. Bradley, Hendricks, and Kabell (2012) and Pope and Vasquez (2011) provide suggestions for what should be covered in this document. According to Pope and Vasquez, issues and questions to consider including in this document are: (a) who will take charge in case of incapacitation or death; (b) who will serve as a backup; (c) the need for coordinated planning should the designee have to take over the practice; (d) making arrangements for access to the office, records, computer systems, your schedule, and client records; (e) direction on how to notify clients and former clients; (f) direction on how to notify colleagues; (g) contact information for the clinician's liability insurance carrier; (h) access to billing records with instruction how to proceed forward; and (i) instructions on paying expenses that may still be due.

Pope and Vasquez further suggest that the document be reviewed by an attorney, that copies be provided to those who are going to execute the will, and that mental health professionals periodically review and update the document. Ballard (2005) emphasizes the need to have a statement in the document providing authorization for the professional executor to implement and follow the directives of the clinician.

BUSINESS ISSUES

In addition to the clinical issues discussed in this chapter, when a practice closes there may still be financial or regulatory issues that require attention. The extent of this depends on the organizational structure of the practice, as there may be different requirements for a sole proprietorship practice as opposed to one that is incorporated.

Zuckerman (2008) presents an excellent "Financial and Contractual Obligations" checklist that outlines many important issues and tasks to be planned for with the closing (expected or unexpected) of a practice. These include (a) meeting with your professional team (attorney, CPA, financial planner) to review procedures and obligations; (b) making arrangements for obligations regarding lease and rental agreements; (c) reviewing the necessary procedures and devising a plan for the dissolution of the corporate entity; (d) developing a plan to arrange for the disposal of tangible assets; (e) developing a plan to deal with outstanding accounts payable and accounts receivable; (f) creating a plan to pay necessary taxes due, as well as other regulatory premiums such as unemployment compensation and workers compensation; and (g) for psychologists, making a plan for ethical disposal or transfer of psychological tests. Following these procedures will go a long way toward reducing the chaos or financial hardship for family members that may ensue following incapacitation or death of the practitioner, as well as fulfilling legal and ethical requirements and obligations.

ETHICAL CHALLENGES

- When you leave a group practice, there may be conflicts between your duty to the welfare of your clients and the contract that you have in place.
- When closing a practice, the primary obligation is to the welfare of clients, regardless of economic implications for the practitioner.
- Some clinicians may choose to maintain therapeutic contact with a client via tele-health modalities after relocating to another jurisdiction. There are legal and ethical issues to consider in providing such services.

- Clients have a right to be involved in decisions regarding any future care they may receive.
- Clients have a right to access their medical records even though their clinician is no longer in practice.
- When selling a practice, protecting client confidentiality and respecting each client's autonomy and right to decide if they wish to continue treatment with the buyer of the practice is paramount.
- Even upon retirement or death, there is an ongoing obligation to former clients.

KEY POINTS TO KEEP IN MIND

- All practices come to an end, whether planned or unplanned.
- You may have obligations to your practice group to meet when leaving the practice.
- The closing of a practice requires paying attention to many details related to clients, practice associates, and business and legal issues.
- You must develop a plan for when to inform clients and referral partners about the closing of the practice.
- In addition to telling current clients, you must inform former clients that the practice is closing.
- Clients may choose to continue with the buyer of a practice or may choose not to do so. They are not the property of the clinician and need to make autonomous decisions about future care.
- Responsibility for past professional behavior does not end when the clinician closes a practice.
- Upon your retirement or death, ethical, legal, or contractual obligations may remain in effect that may fall upon you or your estate.

PRACTICAL RECOMMENDATIONS

- When signing a contract to join a practice, pay special attention to practical, ethical, and legal issues that concern leaving the practice.
- Where possible, plan the closing of the practice, allowing enough time to meet ethical and legal requirements.
- Allow a reasonable amount of time for clients to emotionally process the closing of the practice.
- Be knowledgeable of both ethical and legal obligations for closing a practice.
- Develop a termination of practice letter to be provided to current and former clients, advising them of what is taking place and providing information that will be important to them regarding their records and future care.

- Provide a list of possible referral sources for current and past clients.
- Arrange for record storage and processing for the legally required period of time following the closure of the practice.
- If selling a practice, try to find a buyer with similar practice specialty areas.
- Maintain malpractice insurance several years into retirement and consider purchasing a tail for future protection for past acts where a claim may be made.
- Develop a professional practice will and periodically review it to see if updates are necessary.

PITFALLS TO AVOID

- Assuming contract clauses will not be enforced or litigated when you leave the practice.
- Not planning for what happens to your practice after you die, and having the attitude, "Well, I'll be gone, so why should I care?"
- Assuming clients will be unaffected by the termination of therapy because they are being transferred to another clinician.
- Assuming there is a low likelihood of being caught when providing tele-health services, so there is no need to follow ethical or legal requirements.
- Assuming that treatment records belong to the clinician and that clients have no right to confidentiality of those records or no right to access them.

RELEVANT ETHICS CODE STANDARDS

Telling Clients That You Will No Longer Be Practicing

- AAMFT Code of Ethics (AAMFT, 2012) Principle 1.07, No Furthering of Own Interests, states, "Marriage and family therapists do not use their professional relationships to further their own interests" (p. 2).
- ACA Code of Ethics (ACA, 2005) Standard A.1.a, Primary Responsibility, states, "The primary responsibility of counselors is to respect the dignity and to promote the welfare of clients" (p. 4).
- APA Ethics Code (APA, 2010) Standard 3.08, Exploitive Relationships, states, "Psychologists do not exploit persons over whom they have supervisory, evaluative or other authority such as clients/patients, students, supervisees, research participants and employees" (p. 6).
- NASW Code of Ethics (NASW, 2008) Standard 1.01, Commitment to Clients, states, "Social workers' primary responsibility is to promote the wellbeing of clients. In general, clients' interests are primary" (p. 5).

Maintenance of Records

- AAMFT Code of Ethics (AAMFT, 2012) Principle 2.5, Preparation for Practice Changes, states, "In preparation for moving from the area, closing a practice, or death, marriage and family therapists arrange for the storage, transfer, or disposal of client records in conformance with applicable laws and in ways that maintain confidentiality and safeguard the welfare of clients" (p. 3).
- ACA Code of Ethics (ACA, 2005) Standard B.6.g, Storage and Disposal After Termination, states, "Counselors store records following termination of services to ensure reasonable future access, maintain records in accordance with state and federal statutes governing records, and dispose of client records and other sensitive materials in a manner that protects client confidentiality" (p. 8).
- APA Ethics Code (APA, 2010) Standard 6.02c states, "Psychologists make plans in advance to facilitate the appropriate transfer and to protect the confidentiality of records and data in the event of psychologists' withdrawal from positions or practice" (p. 9).
- NASW Code of Ethics (NASW, 2008) Standard 1.07n, Privacy and Confidentiality, states, "Social workers should transfer or dispose of clients' records in a manner that protects clients' confidentiality and is consistent with state statues governing records and social work licensure" (p. 3).

Selling of a Practice

- AAMFT Code of Ethics (AAMFT, 2010) Principle 2.2, Written Authorization to Release Confidential Information, states, "Marriage and family therapists do not disclose client confidences except by written authorization, or waiver" (p. 2).
- ACA Code of Ethics (ACA, 2005) Standard B.1.c, Respect for Confidentiality, states, "Counselors do not share confidential information without client consent or without sound legal or ethical justification" (p. 7). Further, ACA Ethics Code Standard A.1.a states, "The primary responsibility of counselors is to respect the dignity and to promote the welfare of clients" (p. 4).
- APA Ethics Code (2010) Standard 4.01, Maintaining Confidentiality, states, "Psychologists have a primary obligation and take reasonable precautions to protect confidential information obtained through or stored in any medium, recognizing that the extent and limits of confidentiality may be regulated by law or established through institutional rules or professional or scientific relationship" (p. 7). Further, APA Ethics Code Standard 3.06, Conflicts of Interest, states, "Psychologists refrain from taking on a professional role when personal, scientific, professional, legal, financial,

or other interests or relationships could reasonably be expected to impair
their objectivity, competence, or effectiveness in performing their functions
as psychologists" (p. 6).

- NASW Code of Ethics (NASW, 2008) Standard 1.07, Privacy and
  Confidentiality, states, "Social workers should protect the confidentiality
  of all information in the course of professional service, except for
  compelling professional reasons" (p. 7). Further, NASW Code of
  Ethics Standard 1.01 states, "Social workers' primary responsibility is
  to promote the well-being of clients. In general, clients' interests are
  primary" (p. 2).

The Professional Practice Will

- AAMFT Code of Ethics (AAMFT, 2012) Principle 1.11,
  Non-Abandonment, states, "Marriage and family therapists do not
  abandon or neglect clients in treatment without making reasonable
  arrangements for the continuation of treatment" (p. 3).
- ACA Code of Ethics (ACA, 2005) Standard C.2.h, Counselor
  Incapacitation or Termination of Practice, states, "Counselors prepare and
  disseminate to an identified colleague or 'records custodian' a plan for the
  transfer of clients and files in the case of their incapacitation, death, or
  termination of practice" (p. 10).
- APA Ethics Code (APA, 2010) Standard 3.12, Interruption of Psychological
  Services, states, "Unless otherwise covered by contract, psychologists
  make reasonable efforts to plan for facilitating services in the event that
  psychological services are interrupted by factors such as the psychologist's
  illness, death, unavailability, relocation or retirement" (p. 6).
- NASW Code of Ethics (NASW, 2008) Standard 1.15, Interruption of
  Services, states, "Social workers should make reasonable efforts to ensure
  continuity of services in the event that services are interrupted by factors
  such as unavailability, relocation, illness, disability, or death" (p. 4).

REFERENCES

American Association for Marriage and Family Therapy. (2012). *Code of ethics*. Retrieved
    from http://www.aamft.org/imis15/content/legal_ethics/code_of_ethics.aspx
American Counseling Association. (2005). *ACA code of ethics*. Retrieved from http://
    www.counseling.org/Resources/aca-code-of-ethics.pdf
American Psychological Association. (2010). *Ethical principles of psychologists and code
    of conduct*. Retrieved from http://www.apa.org/ethics

Ballard, D. (2005). Planning ahead to close or sell your practice. In J. E. Barnett & M. Gallardo (Eds.), *Handbook for success in independent practice* (pp. 165–172). Phoenix, AZ: Psychologists in Independent Practice.

Barnett, J. E. (1997). Leaving a practice: Ethical and legal dilemmas. In L. VandeCreek, S. Knapp, & T. Jackson (Eds.), *Innovations in clinical practice* (pp. 181–188). Sarasota, FL: Professional Resource Exchange.

Bennett, B. E., Bricklin, P. M., Harris, E., Knapp, S., VandeCreek, L., & Younggren, J. N. (2006). *Assessing and managing risk in psychological practice: An individualized approach*. Rockville, MD: The Trust.

Bradley, L. J., Hendricks, B., & Kabell, D. R. (2012). The professional will: An ethical responsibility. *The Family Journal, 20*, 309–314.

Harris, E., & Younggren, J. (2012). Visions for the future of professional psychology: Risk management in the digital world. *Professional Psychology: Research and Practice, 43*, 613–621.

Koocher, G. (2003). Ethical and legal issues in professional psychology transitions. *Professional Psychology: Research and Practice, 34*, 383–387.

Manosevitz, M., & Hays, K. (2003). Relocating your psychotherapy practice: Packing and unpacking. *Professional Psychology: Research and Practice, 34*, 375–382.

McGee, T. (2003). Observations on the retirement of professional psychologists. *Professional Psychology: Research & Practice, 34*, 388–395.

National Association of Social Workers. (2008). *Code of ethics*. Retrieved from http://www.socialworkers.org/pubs/code/code.asp

Pope, K. S., & Vasquez, M. J. T. (2011). *Ethics in psychotherapy and counseling: A practical guide* (4th ed.). New York, NY: Wiley.

Walfish, S., & Barnett, J. E. (2009). *Financial success in mental health practice: Essential tools and strategies for practitioners*. Washington, DC: APA Books.

Walfish, S., & Zimmerman, J. (2013). Making good referrals. In G. Koocher, J. Norcross, & B. Greene (Eds.), *Psychologists desk reference* (3rd ed., pp. 649–653). New York, NY: Oxford University Press.

Weitz, R. D., & Samuels, R. M. (1990). The sale and purchase of a private health-service-provider psychology practice. In E. Margeanau (Ed.), *The encyclopedic handbook of private practice* (pp. 384–390). New York, NY: Gardner Press.

Woody, R. H. (1997). Valuing a psychological practice. *Professional Psychology: Research and Practice, 28*, 77–80.

Zuckerman, E. L. (2008). *The paper office* (4th ed). New York, NY: Guilford Press.

10

Closing Thoughts

The development of ethical sensitivities is a process that will span your career and change over time. Years ago there was no need to consider tele-health, security of electronic records, or social media. Looking forward it is difficult to predict the ethical dilemmas you will face in practice, except to say that they will continue to confront you. You will need to respond to these dilemmas by considering client welfare and then behaviorally implementing solutions in a way that allows them to be integrated both clinically and administratively into your practice patterns.

Many times there will not be a single right or wrong answer, but rather the need to weigh many different factors specific to the demands and challenges of the situation before you. By seeking the input of mentors and colleagues, getting the necessary training, and continuing to focus on the nuances of the ethical dilemmas and challenges you encounter, you can make sure you are doing your best to avoid ethical transgressions and mishaps.

We hope this book is a step in the right direction for you, and that you return to it from time to time for input as situations arise over the lifetime of your practice. We wish you the best of luck in developing a clinically sound, financially solid, and ethically based private practice.

ABOUT THE AUTHORS

Jeffrey E. Barnett, PsyD, ABPP, is Professor and Associate Chair in the Department of Psychology at Loyola University Maryland and the Director of Practitioner Master's Programs there. For the past 29 years he has maintained a private practice near Annapolis, Maryland. He is a licensed psychologist and a Diplomate of the American Board of Professional Psychology (ABPP) in Clinical Psychology and in Clinical Child and Adolescent Psychology. Additionally, he is a Distinguished Practitioner of Psychology in the National Academies of Practice and a Fellow of five divisions of the American Psychological Association (APA). Dr. Barnett is a Past President of the Maryland Psychological Association and of three divisions of the APA, and he is a past chair of the APA Ethics Committee. Presently, he is the Vice Chair of the Maryland Board of Examiners of Psychologists and Vice Chair of the ABPP Ethics Committee.

Dr. Barnett has numerous publications and presents regularly on ethical, legal, and professional practice issues for mental health professionals. His recent books include *Billing and Collecting for Your Mental Health Practice* (2011, APA Books; with Steve Walfish), *Ethics Desk Reference for Counselors* (2010, ACA Books; with Brad Johnson), *Ethics Desk Reference for Psychologists* (2008, APA Books; with Brad Johnson), and *Financial Success in Mental Health Practice* (2009, APA Books; with Steve Walfish). Dr. Barnett's areas of professional interest include ethics and professional issues for mental health professionals and trainees, such as self-care and psychological wellness, mentoring, advocacy, leadership, business success in practice and entrepreneurship, and the roles of technology and social media in practice. He has received numerous awards in recognition of his contributions to the profession of psychology, including the 2009 APA Award for Distinguished Contributions to the Independent Practice of Psychology, the 2011 APA Outstanding Ethics Educator Award, and the 2011 Award for Outstanding Contributions to Teaching and Mentoring from APA's Division 29 (Psychotherapy). His CV can be accessed at http://www.loyola.edu/academic/psychology/faculty-staff/faculty/barnett.aspx.

Jeffrey Zimmerman, PhD, ABPP, is a licensed psychologist (Connecticut and New York) and has been in independent practice for over 30 years. He returned to solo practice in 2007 after serving as founding and managing partner of a group practice for 22 years. He has two niche specialty practices (alternative dispute resolution for divorce and organizational consultation) in addition to a general practice where he specializes in the treatment of anxiety, depression, and conflict around divorce. He has also coauthored (with Dr. Elizabeth Thayer) *The Co-Parenting Survival Guide: Letting Go of Conflict After a Difficult Divorce* and *Adult Children of Divorce: How to Overcome the Legacy of Your Parents' Breakup and Enjoy Love, Trust, and Intimacy.* Dr. Zimmerman is also a founding partner of The Practice Institute, LLC. Since 1988 he has been an Assistant Clinical Professor at the Department of Psychiatry, School of Medicine, University of Connecticut, Farmington.

Dr. Zimmerman received his doctorate in clinical psychology from the University of Mississippi (1980). Dr. Zimmerman is a Past President of the Connecticut Psychological Association (1993–1994). In 1997 he became a Fellow of the Connecticut Psychological Association. In 2004 he received the award for Distinguished Contributions to the Practice of Psychology from the Connecticut Psychological Association. In 2009 Dr. Zimmerman received the ABPP specialty board certification in clinical psychology. In 2010 Dr. Zimmerman was made a Fellow of Division 42 (Psychologists in Independent Practice) of the APA in recognition of outstanding contributions to the profession of psychology. In 2011 he was made a Fellow of APA Division 29 (Psychotherapy).

Steven Walfish, PhD, is a licensed psychologist and has been in independent practice in Atlanta since 2002. He is also a founding partner of The Practice Institute, LLC. He received his PhD in clinical/community psychology from the University of South Florida in 1981. He has previously been in independent practice in Tampa, Florida and in Edmonds and Everett, Washington. He has been the Editor of the *Independent Practitioner* and has served on the editorial boards of several journals. He has published in the areas of substance abuse, weight loss surgery, and professional training and practice. He is currently a Clinical Assistant Professor, Department of Psychiatry and Behavioral Sciences, Emory University School of Medicine, where he supervises postdoctoral fellows.

He is recipient of the APA Division of Consulting Psychology Award for Outstanding Research in Consulting Psychology, the Walter Barton Award for Outstanding Research in Mental Health Administration from the American College of Mental Health Administration, and the APA Division of Independent Practice Award for Mentoring. He is a Fellow of APA Division 42 (Psychologists in Independent Practice) and the Georgia Psychological Association, and he is Past President of APA Division 42.

His first book (coedited with Allen Hess) was *Succeeding in Graduate School: The Career Guide for Psychology Students.* His recent books include *Financial Success in Mental Health Practice: Essential Tools and Strategies for Practitioners* (with Jeff Barnett), *Earning a Living Outside of Managed Mental Health Care: 50 Ways to Expand Your Practice, Billing and Collecting for Your Mental Health Practice: Effective Strategies and Ethical Practice* (with Jeff Barnett), and *Translating Psychological Research Into Practice* (coedited with Lisa Grossman).

Note: Page numbers followed by *t* indicate a table on the corresponding page

testimonial endorsements, 137–139
  potential impact on the public, 143
  precautions regarding use of, 141, 144, 145
  relevant ethics code standards, 147
Thomas, J., 5
Turchik, J. A., 113

U.S. Department of Health & Human Services, 110–111

Value Options (MCO), 103

VandeCreek, L., 93
vicarious traumatization, 153

wait time and waiting lists, 30–31
Walfish, S., 14–15, 16, 17, 28, 29, 93, 98–99, 111
wellness, promotion of, 44, 154–155

Younggren, J. N., 93, 99, 166–167

Zimmerman, J., 80–81
Zuckerman, E. L., 163, 164, 167–168

CPSIA information can be obtained
at www.ICGtesting.com
Printed in the USA
BVHW031342140720
583709BV00004B/297

9 780199 976621